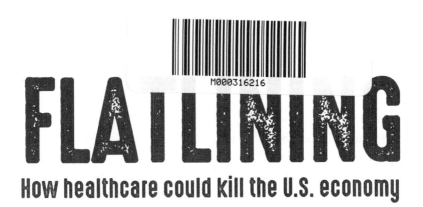

FLATLINING

How healthcare could kill the U.S. economy

RON HOWRIGON

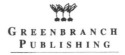

GREENBRANCH
PUBLISHING

Early Praise

"Mr. Howrigon's book offers up a concise healthcare landscape analysis with common-sense treatment recommendations. His extensive and practical career experience representing payers, health systems, and physician practices provides him with a unique and central perspective as an analyst, negotiator, and commentator."

ROBERT E. SCHAAF, MD, FACR
Former President & Managing Partner, Wake Radiology and
Past President of the North Carolina Medical Society

"*Flatlining* is a book that should be read by every person, expert or not, who is interested in healthcare. Ron Howrigon sees healthcare in all its crazy complexity through many vantage points and makes this both fact-based and a good read. I have had the pleasure of working with Ron over the years and he is the real deal."

BOB GRECZYN
CEO Emeritus, BCBSNC

"Ron was the first insurance representative I negotiated against when I became CEO of Raleigh Neurology Associates. Shortly thereafter, we became friends. Then Ron changed sides and became a contract negotiator for providers. That change has been one of two defining moments in the great history of our company. Ron's knowledge of payers and providers is unsurpassed and his insights are invaluable."

STEPHEN M. SMITH, CEO
Raleigh Neurology Associates

"*Flatlining* is an insightful and thought-provoking look at the past, present, and future of healthcare in America."

DONALD GINTZIG,
Rear Admiral USN, Retired, CEO, WakeMed Health and Hospitals

Greenbranch Publishing books are available at special quantity discounts for bulk purchases as premiums, fund-raising, or educational use. info@greenbranch.com or (800) 933-3711.

13   8 7 6 5 4 3 2 1

Copyedited, typeset, and printed in the United States of America

PUBLISHER
Nancy Collins

EDITORIAL ASSISTANT
Jennifer Weiss

COVER DESIGN
Johannah Sloop

BOOK DESIGN
Laura Carter
Carter Publishing Studio
www.carterpublishingstudio.com

COPYEDITOR
Pat George

Table of Contents

Acknowledgments

Every book has a name on the cover for the author. This book has my name on it. In reality there should be a whole list of names on the cover. This book could never have happened without a group of incredible people. While I can't fit all of their names on the cover, I can take this opportunity to thank them here.

First, I would like to thank and acknowledge my team at Fulcrum Strategies. I am very fortunate in that I get to work with the best group of people I have ever known. Each of them challenges, teaches, and inspires me every day. They all have talents and skills that I do not posses. They form the kind of team that most people dream of but never experience. So, I would like to thank Dustin Clark, Kristina Alexander, Ashley Elmore, Trista Nelson, Amy Sink, Johannah Sloop, and Cindy Nyberg. Each of them has in their own way made this book possible and without them none of this would have happened. Thank you all for being the reason I get up every morning and look forward to going to work.

I would like to thank my clients—the physicians all across this country who don't look at healthcare as a policy problem or an economic issue. Instead, they live it every day when they walk into an exam room or an operating room or when they study an image looking for a diagnosis to a patient problem. These are the people on the front line of healthcare who see patients every day who look to them for answers to what often are life's biggest issues and problems. Each of you has my undying respect and my commitment to do whatever I can to help.

Thanks to Nancy Collins and the publishing professionals at Greenbranch Publishing. This book made it from manuscript to finished product in record time. We are proud of the finished book and are grateful for the attention to detail and publishing acumen from the Greenbranch team.

Finally, I would like to thank my wife. She is my balance and my center. She is always there to support me and ground me. No matter what the challenge or the issue, I always know that she will be there as my true north, to keep me balanced with what really matters in life, which is my family. Thank you.

There is a long list of people who also deserve thanks and recognition, but if I listed them all, this part of the book would be longer than the rest and inevitably I would leave someone out. So, rather than kill more trees I will just say: you know who you are and I hope you know how thankful I am for your help, support, and friendship.

About the Author

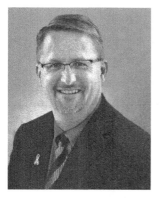

Ron Howrigon is President and Founder of Fulcrum Strategies, based in Raleigh, North Carolina. His experience includes working for several of the largest insurance companies in the country, senior management in a large vertically integrated system, medical practice management and consulting engagements working with thousands of physicians across the country. He has truly seen the full gambit of healthcare delivery and financing scenarios in this country. Ron has "been there and done that." He was awarded a Bachelors in Business Administration with a concentration in Economics from Western Michigan University and a Masters of Economics from North Carolina State University.

In 2004, he founded Fulcrum Strategies to provide contract negotiation services to physicians across the country. The company has grown into offering consulting services including marketing, strategic planning, merger and speaking services to physicians and other related companies.

Ron lives in North Carolina with his wife and three children. His oldest child has Autism which Ron describes as being the hardest and best thing he has ever—or will ever do. Ron is active in his community having served on the Board of Directors for the Mariposa School for Autism and, more recently, the Miracle League of the Triangle, a baseball league dedicated to providing children with special needs the opportunity to participate in an activity that would otherwise not be available to them.

You can contact Ron at r.howrigon@fsdoc.com.

Foreword

Ron Howrigon, has been one of the great professors in my life. As physicians, we naturally have an inclination to constantly learn and consume knowledge. Appropriately, we deeply appreciate those special few who open doors of understanding in areas that are intellectually foggy to us, or for which we never even realized existed.

As a teacher of the business of medicine, Ron has been indispensable in my almost 20-year journey into the process of managing the business of our anesthesia practice. Ron opened the door to the economics of healthcare and helped me understand that the financing of healthcare is an essential component of care delivery in which physicians must participate. It was through Ron's vision and acclimation of our anesthesia practice's strategic positioning years ago to embrace evidence-based medicine and value-based care that our practice moved ahead of the curve in instituting those cutting-edge policies.

The evolution and embracement of evidence-based care and a value-based model have assisted us, and will continue to assist us, in maintaining our independence as practitioners and, more importantly, constantly improving the care of our patients.

The adage, that physicians should focus their energies and attention only on medical practice and leave the financial piece of healthcare to others is, in my opinion, one of the reasons American healthcare has many of the issues it currently has. Medical school education would be greatly enhanced if it required courses taught by Ron on healthcare structure, delivery systems, and finance.

Physicians should participate in the economics of healthcare delivery with as much energy as we contribute clinically, because we are strategically positioned to assist in making the tough choices that the reality of healthcare delivery necessitates. Ron is one of those indispensable partners because of his comprehensive and nuanced understanding of our system, which can facilitate physicians' contributions in the world of medical economics.

If our country is to develop a more successful healthcare future, physicians need to be a major part of the organizational and financial solution. Their participation will simultaneously allow doctors to maintain independence. Independent physicians are more nimble and positioned better to offer solutions. With partners like Ron Howrigon offering advice and guidance, doctors can take on the added responsibilities of global healthcare delivery decision making.

Beyond the primordial call to serve, to do something purposeful in life, the intellectual stimulation of the science of medicine, the requirement for life-long learning, was and still is a great attraction of a physician's professional life. Physicians usually are in love with the practice of medicine. Our commitment to patients is the essential driving force in our existence. Almost universally, physicians, as much as it is humanly possible, will serve and protect our patients against any negative entity. The patient-physician relationship is one of the cornerstones of the great American healthcare community. Because of the desire to do our best, almost all physicians strive to keep expanding our knowledge. We love to learn and problem solve.

Going forward, the paradigm must shift to far greater physician cooperation in shaping healthcare policy if we are to maintain the quality, access, and value our patients have come to expect. My recommendation to those of us willing to take on this challenge, to learn, to participate, to help secure the independent physician-patient model, to make healthcare produce greater value with increased access, is to make Ron's book required reading on the journey.

FRANCIS J. STRANICK, M.D.
Assistant Vice President of Business Development
Providence Anesthesiology Associates

Introduction

When I read a nonfiction or industry-evaluation book, my first thought is about the author. The question that runs through my mind is: what makes him or her an expert in this field? Why would I read any further? What experience and education does he or she have? What point of view does the author bring to this discussion?

I will be the first to admit that there are scores of people who have a more in-depth knowledge of any one sector of healthcare than I possess. However, I believe few people have the same breadth of experience and mix of education that I have accumulated. In 1987 I was awarded a bachelor's of business administration with a concentration in economics from Western Michigan University. And, at the age of 21, began my career in healthcare when I took a job as a medical economics analyst for Kaiser Permanente's North Carolina Health Plan.

Kaiser had begun enrolling their first members on January 1, 1985. I joined Kaiser Permanente on July 1, 1987 as the health plan's 35th employee. At that point I knew absolutely nothing about healthcare.

Early in my employment at Kaiser, I was involved with the numbers side of healthcare. My analysis helped determine our premium rates and the costs for benefit adjustments to our core plans. I learned how offered benefits and employer contributions affected the final insurance premium. I also was involved with make/buy financial analysis. Kaiser continued to struggle with the balance between the "Kaiser model," where everything was done in one of our facilities, and the independent practice association (IPA) model, where care was provided via contract with a community physician or hospital.

I helped run the analysis to determine how our network would be built. Which specialty physicians and services would we add to our own Kaiser medical offices? Which ones would we purchase from the community? Was it more cost-effective to own a CT machine or purchase those scans from community providers? That's when I learned clinical need isn't the only driving factor behind the rate of utilization for many services.

After a few years as an analyst, I was promoted to contract negotiator in the Community Medical Services Department. This department was responsible for negotiating contracts with outside physicians and hospitals for the services we either couldn't, or simply didn't, provide ourselves. Here, I was exposed not only to the business side of the delivery of healthcare in this country, but also to the medical community's general disdain for managed care.

During one of my early hospital negotiations, my boss and I were trying to "educate" the CEO of a local hospital as to the value of a relationship with Kaiser. We kept talking about how Kaiser does things in California and why that approach would help the people of North Carolina. After some time, the hospital CEO brought out a map of the United States. He circled California and then said; "California!" He then circled the rest of the country and said; "NOT California!" This was my first lesson in the truism that all healthcare is local. What was working in California was clearly not going to work in North Carolina.

While working at Kaiser Permanente, I enrolled in a graduate program at North Carolina State University and in 1991 was awarded a master's degree in economics with a minor in statistics. I believed, and still do, that understanding the principles of macro- and micro-economics is the key to understanding how healthcare works.

I also think it's the key to fixing the issues we have with what has become the largest single sector of the U.S. economy.

After spending eight years working for Kaiser Permanente of North Carolina I accepted a position with Cigna HealthCare in their Utah

Health Plan. This was my first experience working for a publicly traded, for-profit company and a pure IPA-model health plan. I spent two and a half years with the Utah Health Plan and then transferred to New Mexico as the executive director of the Lovelace Health Plan for Cigna. Lovelace was one of the few fully integrated health plans and delivery systems in the country and was the only one Cigna owned.

My time at Lovelace showed me the complexities and inherent conflicts of interest involved in the healthcare system. It also was my first foray into managed Medicaid, as I was involved with New Mexico's transition from a traditional Medicaid model to a managed Medicaid model under Governor Gary Johnson.

After a short stint at Lovelace I transferred back to North Carolina to take over Network Management and Contracting for the North Carolina health plan. Eventually South Carolina, Kentucky, Tennessee and Arkansas were added to my territory. This was shortly after Cigna acquired Healthsource, a local payer that operated in North and South Carolina. My first job was to merge not only the provider networks, but also the Cigna and Healthsource staff members. I got to see first-hand what happens after payer consolidation occurs and how it impacts the providers of care and the contracts they hold with insurance companies.

The final stop in my journey working for the payers was at Capital BlueCross in Pennsylvania. I had grown a bit disillusioned with the for-profit, Wall Street-brand of payer environment and decided to go to a nonprofit, independent Blue Cross plan. I thought what was bothering me about working for the payers in general was the pressure of performing to external expectations and trying to please the market's desire for higher and higher stock prices.

After only 12 months as vice president of network management for Capital Blue Cross in Harrisburg, I realized that many of the things I found concerning working for payers were present in the nonprofit world as well and had nothing to do with Wall Street pressures. That's when I made the biggest change—and took the largest risk of my life.

At 39 years old, I started my own consulting company. I began Fulcrum Strategies with the idea that I wanted to try to help physicians navigate the very complex payer environment that I had been working in for almost two decades. I started by representing physician groups in their negotiations with managed care companies, but along the way and over the last 12 years, I have also been the COO of a large specialty group, developed physician compensation models, worked in a small niche lab company, worked for some big pharma companies, and assisted several groups with strategic planning and mergers. Recently I have been doing work in an ACO, clinically integrated network, and value-based reimbursement models.

I have the perspective of a small employer that offers health insurance to its employees. I sign the check every month to pay the premiums for my employees. A check that every month is second only to payroll. I have personally felt the impact of the Affordable Care Act when its changes to underwriting rules sent my premiums ratcheting up over 30% in one year. This increase to expense to my business caused me not to replace an employee who left the company to move to another city. That's one job lost just to pay for an increase in the cost of healthcare.

Finally, I am the father of a child with autism. Most of my son's therapy and treatments are not covered by insurance. I live the very real dilemma of having a family member who needs medical care that isn't "covered." I understand the challenges and burden that situation can place on a family.

I hope the following pages make you think about this important topic, but more importantly, I hope they help you prepare for the tectonic shifts in healthcare and the economy in our future.

CHAPTER 1

The Economics of Healthcare

"Truth is like poetry. Unfortunately, most people hate poetry."

This is a quote from the movie "The Big Short," a movie about the collapse of the housing market in 2007 and 2008 and the few people who actually saw it coming. A fair amount of the movie is dedicated to the resistance of almost everyone else—including the government, the banking industry, and the financial markets—to recognize the truth that the housing bubble was going to collapse.

Truth can be a very difficult thing to handle. This book deals with some difficult truths in a very open and honest way. Some truths, like "We cannot provide everything to everyone. Rationing will happen," are difficult to accept when you're talking about healthcare. Even so, we need to deal with these truths. If we don't, the crash of the health-care market will make the housing crash look like a minor hiccup.

So, if you don't like the poetry of truth, you should probably put this book down and lose yourself in some good fiction. Maybe pick up the latest Grisham novel? If, on the other hand, you are concerned about the direction of our healthcare system and the effect it could have on our economy, please keep reading.

HEALTHCARE

To begin to understand the business of healthcare and how it's likely to change in the future, it's helpful to start with a brief lesson in economics. We begin with a common understanding of microeconomic principles and how they do, or in some cases specifically don't, relate to healthcare.

MICROECONOMICS

The basic principle behind microeconomic theory is the study of *human behavior*. Economists try to explain human behavior in terms of economic activities. When they understand why and how humans engage in economic activities and transactions, they then use that understanding to model and predict human behaviors in various situations. One of the cornerstone concepts is that humans will in most situations act in their own best self-interest. Another basic building block is that humans place their own value on things and that different people may value the same thing differently. Understanding these two concepts helps define how markets work and why they work.

For example, I am a car enthusiast. My wife would call me a "car nut" but I like the term "enthusiast." When I see a rare or old car I place a certain internal value on that car. My wife on the other hand would place a significantly lower value on the same item. Other people like me may place a similar internal value on that car and some may value it even more than I do. Because of this, the price that a particular car could be sold for is a function of its value to a potential buyer. While we use currency as our measure of value, what we're really doing is trading a certain amount of personal *work* for that vehicle.

Economists know that determining the price of a product or service is more complicated than just looking at the value individuals place on that product. They must factor in the relationship between the amount of that product or service available to be purchased (supply) compared to the amount of that product or service people want to buy (demand). This concept of *supply and demand* is especially relevant to healthcare.

Let's take my car example again. Say there are two people in the world who are interested in buying a particular kind of car and both of them are at an auction. What happens if there are three cars of that type being auctioned? When the first one comes up it will sell to the person who places the highest value on it. The second car will be sold to the other person in the audience who wants one, probably for a similar price. When the third car comes up for auction there is no one left who wants the car badly enough to pay the price the first two cars fetched. If the seller wants to sell that car, he will have to lower the price until he reaches a value that is low enough to attract another buyer. In this scenario, supply exceeds demand and whenever that happens price goes down.

In that same situation, if there were only two cars available and three buyers were present, we would see the opposite effect. Demand would exceed supply and a "bidding war" could start that would drive up prices. This is the basic concept of supply and demand. The only thing you need to understand to move forward is the relationships between supply, demand, and prices. Supply has an inverse relationship to price in that the more supply there is, the lower the price will drop. Demand, on the other hand, has a direct relationship price. The higher the demand for a product or service climbs, the higher the price for that product or service will be.

One more economic principle we need to explore is the idea of *rational purchasing decisions*. Economic theories and modeling at a microeconomic level work only in areas of rational purchasing decisions. Rational purchasing decisions are made without some other factor that would cause the consumer to pay more or less than he otherwise would for a given product or service. The opposite of that is a collector.

Let's say you are a baseball card collector and you need one last card to complete a set. Because it's the last card you need for that set, you may be willing to pay more for that card than it would otherwise be worth. That is an example of an irrational purchasing decision, because the very last card you need makes it worth more *to you* than it would be to anyone else.

Healthcare can, by its very nature, be an emotional decision, and therefore not subject to some of the rational decision-making factors that economists count on in efficient marketplaces. How many people would be willing to use a mediocre surgeon who had a higher chance of a complication to save a little money? Not many. When it comes to healthcare, people often say that "money is no object." They want their loved ones to get "the very best." This is one of the problems with healthcare and helps produce inflationary pressure.

MACROECONOMICS

Ok, let's shift from looking at individuals to looking at the big picture—from micro- to macroeconomics. It's important to understand where healthcare fits into the big picture when it comes to the economy at large. Most people who don't work in the industry don't clearly understand how much of the U.S. economy healthcare makes up. In fact, given the size of the economy, healthcare in the U.S. can be impactful on the *world* economy. This is important to understand because future changes in healthcare not only affect how we get care and how much we pay for it, but could also significantly affect things like unemployment, the national debt, and interest rates. These influences on the U.S. economy will have a ripple effect on other countries around the world.

In 1960, healthcare as a market accounted for only 5% of the U.S. economy. For every dollar transacted, only 5 cents were spent for healthcare. The entire U.S. economy was $543 billion, and healthcare accounted for about $27 billion. By itself, in 1960, the U.S. healthcare market would rank as the 15th largest world economy, putting it just in front of the GDP (Gross Domestic Product) of Australia and just behind the GDP of Italy.

Think about that for a minute: the U.S. spent more money on healthcare than the Australians did on everything! To put this further into perspective, in 1960, the U.S. Department of Defense was twice as large as healthcare. The Defense Department consumed 10% of the U.S. economy, which means it would rank as the 11th largest world economy just in front of Japan and just behind China.

Now fast-forward 50 years.

In 2010, the United States GDP was $15 trillion. The total healthcare expenditures in the United States for 2010 were $2.6 trillion. At $2.6 trillion, the U.S. healthcare market has moved up from 15th and now ranks as the 5th largest world economy, just behind Germany and just ahead of both France and the United Kingdom. That means that while healthcare was only 5% of GDP in 1960, it has risen to over 17% of GDP in only 50 years. Over that same time, the Defense Department has gone from 10% of GDP to less than 5% of GDP. This means that in terms of its portion of the U.S. economy, defense spending has been reduced by half while healthcare spending has more than tripled.

If healthcare continues to trend at the same pace it has for the last 50 years, it will consume more than 50% of the U.S. economy by the year 2060. Every economist worth their salt will tell you that healthcare will never reach 50% of the economy. It's simply not possible because of all the other things it would have to crowd out to reach that point. So, if we know healthcare can't grow to 50% of our economy, where is the breaking point? At what point does healthcare consume so much of the economy that it breaks the bank, so to speak?

This is the big question when it comes to healthcare. If something doesn't happen to reverse the 50-year trend we've been riding, when will the healthcare bubble burst? How bad will it be and how exactly will it happen? While no one knows the exact answers to those questions, economists and healthcare experts agree that something needs to happen, because we simply can't continue on this trend forever.

Another way to look at healthcare is to study its impact on the federal budget and the national debt. In 1998, federal healthcare spending accounted for 19% of the revenue taken in by the government. Just eight years later, in 2006, healthcare spending had increased to 24% of federal revenue. In 2010, the Affordable Healthcare Act passed and significantly increased federal spending for healthcare—so much so that in 2016, healthcare spending accounted for almost one-third of all revenue received by the government and surpassed Social Security as the largest single budget category. What makes this trend even more alarming is the fact that revenue to the federal government *doubled* from 1998 to 2016. That means healthcare spending by the federal government has almost *quadrupled* in terms of actual dollars in that same time period. If this trend continues for the next 20 years, healthcare spending will account for over half the revenue received by the government by the year 2035. Again, that simply can't happen without causing significant issues for the financial wellbeing of our country.

In recent history, the U.S. economy has experienced the near catastrophic failure of two major market segments. The first was the auto industry and the second was the housing industry. While each of these reached their breaking point for different reasons, they both required a significant government bailout to keep them from completely melting down. What is also true about both of those market failures is that, looking back, it's easy to see the warning signs. What happens if healthcare is the next industry to suffer a major failure and collapse?

It's safe to say that a healthcare meltdown would make both the automotive and housing industries' experiences seem minor in comparison. While that may be hard to believe, it becomes clear if you look at the numbers. The auto industry contributes around 3.5% of this country's GDP and employs 1.7 million people. This industry was deemed "too big to fail" which is the rationale the U.S. government used to finance its bail out. From 2009 through 2014, the federal government invested around $80 billion in the U.S. auto industry to keep it from collapsing. Healthcare is five *times* larger than the auto industry in terms of its percentage of GDP, and is *ten times* larger than the auto industry in terms of the number of people it employs.

The construction industry (which includes all construction, not just housing) contributes about 6% of our country's GDP and employs 6.1 million people. Again, the healthcare market dwarfs this industry. It's three times larger in terms of GDP production and, with 18 million people employed in the healthcare sector, it's three times larger than construction in this area, too.

These comparisons give you an idea of just how significant a portion healthcare comprises of the U.S. economy. It also begins to help us understand the impact it would have on the economy if healthcare melted down like the auto and housing industries did. So, let's continue the comparison and use our experience with the auto and housing industries to suggest to what order of magnitude the impact a failure in the healthcare market would cause our economy.

The bailout in the auto industry cost the federal government $80 billion over five years. Imagine a similar failure in healthcare that prompted the federal government to propose a similar bailout program. Let's imagine the government felt the need to inject cash into hospital systems and doctors' offices to keep them afloat like they did with General Motors. Since healthcare is five times the size of the auto industry, a similar bailout could easily cost in excess of $400 billion. That's about the same amount of money the federal government spends on welfare programs. To pay for a bailout of the healthcare industry, we'd have to eliminate *all* welfare programs in this country. Can you imagine the impact it would have on the economy if there were suddenly none of the assistance programs so many have come to rely upon?

When the housing market crashed, it caused the loss of about 3 million jobs from its peak employment level of 7.4 million in 1996. Again, if we transfer that experience to the healthcare market, we come up with a truly frightening scenario. If healthcare lost 40% of its jobs like housing did, it would mean 7.2 million jobs lost. That's more than four times the number of people who are employed by the entire auto industry—an industry that was considered too *big* to be allowed to fail.

The loss of 7.2 million jobs would increase the unemployment rate by 5%. That means we could easily top the all-time high unemployment rate for our country. In November of 1982, the U.S. unemployment rate was 10.8%. A failure in the healthcare sector could push unemployment to those levels or higher. The only time in our country's history when unemployment was higher was during the Great Depression. It should also be noted that in 1982, home mortgage interest rates were close to 20%! The U.S. Federal Funds Rate, or the interest rate the government pays on our national debt, was also close to 20% in 1982.

Economists fear that a large increase in unemployment could cause interest rates to escalate to levels approaching those of the early 1980s. If that were to happen today, with a $19 trillion national debt, it would mean that our annual debt service would be $3.8 trillion. Keep in mind that the federal government only takes in $3.4 trillion in total revenue. That's right, in our nightmare scenario where healthcare fails and eliminates 7.2 million jobs, which pushes unemployment above 10% and causes interest rates to climb to almost 20%, we would be in a situation where the interest payments on our current debt would be more than our entire federal tax revenue. Basically, we would be Greece, but on a much larger scale.

Ok, now it's time to take a deep breath. I'm not convinced that healthcare is fated to unavoidable failure and economic catastrophe. That's a worst-case scenario. The problem is that at even a fraction the severity of the auto or housing industry crises we've already faced, a healthcare collapse would still be devastating. Healthcare can't be allowed to continue its current inflationary trending. I believe we are on the verge of some major changes in healthcare, and that how they're implemented will determine their impact on the overall economic picture in this country and around the world. Continued failure to recognize the truth about healthcare will only cause the resulting market corrections to be worse than they need to be.

I don't want to diminish the pain and anguish that many people caught up in the housing crash experienced. I think an argument can be made, though, that if the healthcare market crashes and millions of people end up with no healthcare, the resulting fallout could be much worse than even the housing crisis.

CHAPTER 2

Follow the Money

Now that we have a good basic understanding of the economics of healthcare, we need to understand how it is financed and where the money goes. In the movie "All the President's Men," the reporters were told to "follow the money" if they wanted to unravel what was going on. That's good advice if you want to understand some of the problems with healthcare and why it's close to a meltdown. So, let's take a little journey and try to understand where almost $3 trillion of our money in this country goes every year. Let's follow the money!

We need to start by identifying the various parties that are actually paying for healthcare in the United States. We also need to understand what portion of that cost is *borrowed*. The first in line are federal and state governments. Their expenses include Medicare, Medicaid, and now, the federal subsidies paid to people who purchase health insurance on one of the Affordable Care Act exchanges. Purchasing by a government entity must be financed through taxes or the creation of debt. Right now, the federal government spends $1.12 trillion a year on healthcare. As we learned earlier, that's almost 30% of total government spending each year.

The states combined spend another $563 billion per year on healthcare. While spending for each state varies greatly, on average, 15% of a state's budget goes to pay for Medicaid and the Children's Health Insurance Program (CHIP). That does not include the money that each state pays for healthcare for its own employees. At 15%, healthcare is the second-largest budget expense behind primary and secondary education—and *in front* of higher education. This state money, too, has to come from taxation or the creation of debt.

Employers pay just under $1 trillion per year on health insurance for their employees. While individual numbers are based on type of employer, size, geographic area, and other factors, on average, health insurance costs account for 7.6% of total employee compensation.

The remaining $300 billion are out-of-pocket expenses paid by healthcare consumers. This includes payments made by those who have no insurance as well as payments for co-pays, deductibles, etc.

So we have three major entities that are financing healthcare in this country: federal and state governments combined finance over half (56%) of all healthcare in this country; employers pay for 34% of the bill; and the remaining 10% is paid by the actual consumers of care. In the end, no matter who pays for it, healthcare creates a burden on the economy. Government payments increase taxes or debt, employers' contributions increase the cost of goods and services, and the consumer's portion reduces disposable income.

The fact that the consumer of the service pays for only a tenth of the cost of the service creates a significant problem with the economics of healthcare. That's one of many reasons for the long-term hyperinflation of healthcare costs in this country. For the most part, the *consumer* of this service (the patient) is not the *purchaser* of the service. Whenever the consumers are mostly insulated from their purchasing decisions they tend to make irrational purchasing decisions. Let's look at it this way. Say that as a benefit, your employer allows you to pick any company car you want and pay only 10% of the cost of the car; your employer will pay the other 90%. What kind of car do you think most people would get? Most people would purchase a more expensive car because they don't have to worry about paying for it. This behavior would drive up the cost of cars, as producers would begin producing more expensive, and likely higher-quality, vehicles.

This is not too dissimilar to what has happened in healthcare over the last several decades. We have made significant advancements in the quality of care that we can provide. We have produced a healthcare delivery system with unparalleled access and major advancements in technology. Part of the reason this has happened is the consumers of all of this improvement are insulated from the price tag that comes with these advancements.

That leads us to our next topic: *What impact has the rising cost of healthcare really had on the average American family?* Any time the cost of a product goes up, it has an impact on the purchasing power of the average American family's paycheck. We understand that if the price of gas goes up, the average American family has less money available to purchase other things. Unless wages also improve, we experience a loss in disposable income. So, the question is: how much has the inflation in healthcare actually cost the average American family?

Recently the Rand Corporation, a well-respected, non-partisan research organization, did a study on this very question. The study revealed some alarming conclusions. The Rand study looked at four areas where the cost of healthcare impacts the average American family:

1. **The impact to the average American family caused by the cost of the employer contribution to healthcare premiums.** The more the employer has to pay for this benefit, the less money available for raises and other forms of compensation or benefits.

2. **The employee contribution.** Increases in the employee contribution to their healthcare are a direct reduction in salary or income.

3. **Out-of-pocket expenses.** Recently we have seen many employers reduce benefits by moving to things like high-deductible plans. This reduction in benefits directly impacts the finances of the average American family.

4. **The portion of taxes that are devoted to healthcare.** Again, governmental purchases of healthcare or individual subsidies for the

Affordable Care Act (ACA) exchanges drive up taxes to finance them.

These four areas make up the total impact of healthcare inflation on the American family.

The study period was from 1999 to 2009. In that decade, the cost of healthcare in this country nearly doubled. It should be noted that the Affordable Care Act didn't pass until 2010, and while many still hope that this legislation will eventually help reduce the cost of healthcare, most people agree that the data from the first few years points to a dramatic *increase* in the cost of care. None of this increase is evaluated in the Rand study. The study points out that almost *all* wage increases for the period were consumed by the increased cost of healthcare. In fact, in 2009, the average American family, after paying for the increased cost of healthcare, was left with only $95 per month of additional income compared to 1999. That's an annual growth rate in income not consumed by healthcare increases of less than $10 per month. After inflation, that means the average American worker has actually lost ground in terms of disposable income after paying for the cost increases in healthcare.

As if that weren't enough, the study goes on to point out that the total picture is even worse. You see, in 1999, the federal budget was balanced. This meant all healthcare costs were covered by either the private or public sector. In 2009, the federal government was running a significant deficit, which means that some portion of healthcare costs were being financed through debt. If the federal government had chosen not to pursue this kind of deficit financing of healthcare and instead increased taxes to cover the real cost of healthcare, the average American family's tax bill would have been $390 per month higher than it was in 1999. Under this scenario, the impact of health-care costs on the average American family wouldn't be a $95 increase in income over the previous decade, but would instead be a $295 per month decrease in income.

Another way to look at things would be to calculate how the average American family would have been positively impacted if healthcare had inflated only at the standard inflation rate (CPI-U) over that decade. In this scenario, the average American family would have experienced an increase in disposable income of $450 per month comparing 2009 to 1999. Imagine what impact an extra $5,000 of disposable income per family could have on the U.S. economy.

Now it's time to look at the impact of healthcare costs on the employers in this country and how it affects their ability to compete in a global economy. Economists agree, market places are becoming ever more global in nature, less restricted by geography every year. More U.S. companies are competing globally for the goods and services they produce. This reality has increased the utilization of outsourcing, overseas production, and off-shore service industries—largely due to the lower cost of doing business in other countries compared to the United States. How many times have you heard a friend or neighbor complain about a product being made in another country, or calling a customer service line only to have it answered by someone who is obviously outside the United States? Unfortunately, it makes financial sense for many U.S. firms to move production or services out of this country. How much of those lower operating costs can be attributed to the cost of healthcare in America? What impact does the rising cost of healthcare have on employers and labor that remain in this country?

Let's begin by looking at healthcare spending per capita and as a percentage of GDP by country. Today the United States spends almost 20% of its GDP on healthcare. That's twice as much as most other industrialized nations. That kind of spending puts a significant strain on the U.S. economy.

In 1970, the United States spent about the same per capita on healthcare as Canada and most of Europe. By 1985, our healthcare inflation had moved us into first place when it comes to per-capita spending. Today the U.S. spends more than twice as much per capita on healthcare as do other similar industrialized nations. It's easy to see from this information the increased pressure that trend puts on U.S. businesses. The longer this trend continues, the more pressure and incentive there will be on U.S. businesses to transfer part, or all, of their operations and production overseas.

The disadvantage carried by U.S. companies is significant. For example, let's once again look at the auto industry. General Motors pays over 50% more for healthcare per worker hour than does Toyota. GM estimates that healthcare costs add over $1,500 to the cost of each car they produce. With GM paying more than 50% more for healthcare than Toyota, almost $1,000 is added to the price of a Chevy that isn't there for a Toyota or a Honda. The base Chevy Malibu lists at $22,500 while the base Toyota Camry has a sticker price that is $23,070, only $570 more than the Chevy. However, if GM paid the same for healthcare as Toyota, the Malibu would hold a $1,570 price advantage over to the Camry. How many more people might choose the Chevrolet over the Toyota at that price point?

A study by the National Bureau of Economic Research examined the impact of rising healthcare costs on the labor market. The study concluded that every 10% increase in healthcare costs decreased the number of paid work hours by 1%—and your chances of *being* employed by 1.6%. This clearly shows the direct correlation of rising healthcare costs to both under- and unemployment. Further, the study concluded that increases in healthcare costs are increasingly being borne by our labor forces in the form of wage reductions. For every 10% increase in healthcare costs, real wages are reduced by 2.3% as employers attempt to offset healthcare increases that, in many cases, cannot be transferred to product price in an increasingly competitive global economy.

Diving deeper into the numbers shows that low-wage, hourly workers are impacted the most by rising healthcare costs. Employers have minimum wage limitations for these workers, so reductions in payroll have to be realized with layoffs or hiring freezes. Many of the businesses in question are small, exempting them from penalties if they decide to drop healthcare coverage entirely.

Arguably, people who fall into this segment of the labor force are the least likely to be able to purchase health insurance on their own, even with the new federal subsidies in the health exchanges. As such, if they're laid off, or their employer suddenly decides to drop their insurance due to the rising costs of providing coverage, these Americans are most likely to go without it.

If we take all of these factors into consideration, it's plain to see the negative impact of rising healthcare costs on our economy. It puts pressure on employers to shift production or service overseas, which increases unemployment. It puts pressure on employers to reduce wages to remain competitive, which decreases disposable income in this country and slows economic growth. Finally, it puts pressure on small employers to reduce or eliminate the healthcare coverage they offer their employees to offset rising costs that can't be pushed to the market through higher pricing.

All of this illustrates the fact that healthcare, as a market segment, is *enormous*. It impacts almost every other segment of our economy. The increase in healthcare costs has had a dramatic impact on government spending, taxes, employers and their employees, and the American family. If we draw these individual pressures and impacts together and look at their impacts in total, several truths stand out from the dire landscape we've revealed:

Truth: The cost of healthcare has been inflating at an unsustainable rate for the last several decades.

Truth: Healthcare costs cannot be allowed to continue to inflate at rates faster than CPI-U.

Truth: If left unchecked, healthcare inflation will result in a market adjustment that could send the U.S. economy into a tailspin, the likes of which we haven't seen since the Great Depression.

These are facts, and as President John Adams once said:

"Facts are stubborn things; and whatever may be our wishes, our inclinations, or the dictates of our passion, they cannot alter the state of facts and evidence."

CHAPTER 3

A Brief History of Healthcare and Insurance in America

For over 100 years after the birth of this nation, healthcare in America was a completely self-pay system. We all have visions of the local country doctor and his black bag making house calls—which were paid for either in cash or by trade. This system worked reasonably well for a century. However, as medicine advanced and the cost of care began to increase, the possibility of a two-tiered system started to become more likely. The wealthy would get care because they could afford the advances—the working class would not.

In 1910, one of the earliest examples of health insurance was created. The Western Clinic in Tacoma, Washington, provided a wide variety of healthcare services to the employees of local lumber mills. The cost was 50 cents per month. In 1929, Dr. Michael Shadid created something similar to the model in Tacoma. Dr. Shadid created a healthcare cooperative in rural Oklahoma where farmers could pay a predetermined monthly fee for which he would provide all of their care. These two early examples were driven by healthcare providers without the middle man—known later as the insurance company.

In 1929, the Ross-Loos Medical Group was established in Los Angeles. The medical group offered its services to county and city employees for a premium of $1.50 per month. Baylor Hospital in Texas started its own plan in 1929 for about 1500 teachers. This plan eventually became what we know now as BlueCross and Blue Shield (BCBS). The seeds of the insurance industry were planted and quickly took root.

In 1933, Dr. Sidney Garfield and several of his associates started another pre-paid care delivery model in southern California. This model contracted with the LA Workers Compensation Insurance companies to care for job site injuries while the workers themselves contributed out of their pocket for routine medical issues. A few years later, Dr. Garfield connected with Henry Kaiser and formed both the Kaiser Foundation Health Plans and the Permanente Medical Group, which many people have come to know as Kaiser Permanente—the first HMO. This development led to an explosion of similar local or regional delivery systems and plans. Group Health Association (GHA), Health Insurance Plan, and Group Health of Puget Sound were all formed during this time frame. In 1933, the first BCBS-covered baby was delivered in Durham, North Carolina. The mother stayed in the hospital for 10 days and the entire hospital bill was $60.

In the 1940s, the country faced a labor shortage brought on by increased factory production and a reduced labor force as many of America's young men went off to fight World War II. The government put into place a number of wage controls. As a result, companies began offering healthcare insurance as a fringe benefit to attract employees. The government wanted to encourage this practice so it offered business income tax exemptions for healthcare-related expenses. These factors gave birth to the development and growth of our current employer-based health insurance model.

In 1965, the federal government enacted legislation that created Medicare and Medicaid to provide coverage for the country's poor and elderly. These programs were thought to provide a solution for the two main groups of people who were not covered by employer-based insurance, namely the unemployed and the elderly who were no longer part of the work force.

In the 1970s, a big push began in this country to address some of the perceived failings of the then-current system. Issues around escalating costs, patient's rights, coverage of the uninsured that didn't qualify for Medicare or Medicaid, and cries for reform brought about the HMO Act of 1973. This act created loans and grants for starting new HMOs or expanding existing ones. The Act also served to override state restrictions on HMOs if the HMO was federally qualified. Finally, the Act required employers with more than 25 employees to offer a federally qualified HMO in addition to the traditional indemnity coverage offered to their employees.

This is important because, while nowhere near as sweeping as the most recent reform legislation, the HMO Act of 1973 did two things that were revolutionary at the time in healthcare, and possibly influenced the shape of our most recent round of reforms. First, the Act allowed the federal government to override state legislation when it came to HMOs. This is particularly interesting when you consider the Supreme Court ruling in 2012 that stated the federal government could *not* force states to expand Medicaid. The waters navigated by the state and federal governments certainly get murky where they mix. The HMO Act was never even challenged in court, though many attorneys considered it a violation of the Commerce Clause—not to mention a gross overstepping of federal authority. It simply passed. The Medicaid expansion, granting similar rights to the federal government over the states, was challenged and struck down by the Supreme Court. There's no clear sailing here.

The other revolutionary aspect of the HMO Act of 1973 is the requirement that employers offer a federally qualified HMO alongside their indemnity coverage. When this was passed in 1973, there was a chorus of employer organizations that argued against the ability and wisdom of the federal government dictating insurance coverage to the business community. There are similar arguments going on today from businesses that claim the government's intrusion into employer-based healthcare is damaging to the economy and their businesses.

Beginning in the 1970s, and continuing through the turn of the century, we witnessed an explosion of HMOs and the expansion of a whole host of insurance products that we now collectively call managed care. This time period also saw healthcare costs continue to inflate faster than general economic growth and faster than government tax revenue growth. Many thought managed care, with its admittedly limited tool bag, would be the answer to controlling medical costs. That HMOs and other network-based insurance products were expanding *while* we were also producing significant increases in the cost of healthcare put the lie to that assumption early on.

In 1992, then-Governor Bill Clinton campaigned heavily on a proposed universal healthcare platform as he pursued and won the presidential election that year. Clinton spoke on many occasions about how millions of Americans were without healthcare and millions more were "just one pink slip away from losing their healthcare" in this country. Once elected, President Clinton set up a task force headed by First Lady Hillary Clinton to develop legislation to produce universal healthcare coverage in the United States. The plan that came out of that task force required employers to provide insurance for their employees and required all Americans to purchase a qualified health plan. It also provided government subsidies so that Americans below a certain income level received their coverage at no cost. At this point, you're probably thinking this sounds suspiciously like what eventually was passed with the Affordable Care Act.

The push for "Hillary Care," as its detractors dubbed the plan, faced opposition not only from the right, but also some on the left who favored a single-payer system rather than a market-based solution with employer and public mandates. A set of TV ads showing a couple sitting at a kitchen table talking about losing their doctor and their choices helped turn the tide against the plan, and finally, in 1994,

Senate Majority Leader George Mitchell declared the bill dead. The first real attempt at modern healthcare reform was defeated.

What's interesting to note is the impact that the threat of reform had on healthcare inflation. If you look at the period from 1980 to 1990, healthcare costs as a percentage of GDP increased by 3.2%. That means that healthcare inflated at a rate that is 3.2% faster than the growth of the economy during that decade. During the decade from 1990 to 2000, which had the threat of Hillary Care, healthcare inflated only 1.2% faster than general economic growth. For the period from 2000 to 2008, after the threat of reform was dismissed, the inflation went back to 2.6% faster than general economic growth. This would suggest the threat of government intervention that scared both the provider and payer segments of healthcare had the effect of diminishing cost increases. As soon as the threat passed, the market went back to its old ways of inflating faster than economic growth could keep up.

In 2008, Illinois Senator Barak Obama ran as the Democratic Party nomination for the presidency of the United States. Like, President Clinton, one of his key platform positions was healthcare reform. Since the last attempt in 1992, healthcare inflation had taken its toll on the U.S. economy. The number of people in this country who were uninsured exceeded 40 million by some accounts. Shortly after assuming office, President Obama, with a majority in the House and Senate, set about developing *and passing* a sweeping healthcare reform bill. Having learned lessons from the last attempt, the president knew that he had to strike quickly, and that if he lost either the House or the Senate in the mid-term elections, his hope for healthcare reform would be gone.

On December 24, 2009, the Senate passed the Patient Protection and Affordable Care Act (ACA) and sent it to the president's desk where it was signed into law in March 2010. This law is the biggest piece of healthcare legislation since the creation of Medicare and

Medicaid in 1965. The law set in motion some tectonic shifts in the healthcare landscape that we are only now beginning to understand some five years later.

The logical question, considering our history, is how did we get *here*? What drove this country and its elected officials to pass massive legislation impacting the largest single segment of the U.S. economy? How does a president and Congress pass a piece of legislation that could not be fully understood by anyone at the time—one that, if it fails, could cause the collapse of an economic market that accounts for over 17% of the U.S. economy? To answer those questions, you need to understand the failures that preceded the passing of the ACA and how those failures, along with several other key factors, turned out to be a perfect storm in political timing.

From the 1980s through the end of the century, the expansion of managed care did many things. It increased the types of products and options that were offered to employers. It increased choice and competition in a market place that just a few decades before had little to none. Managed care introduced a variety of cost controls, some that worked and some that didn't. It also created a financial entity that got in the middle of the doctor and patient relationship in some cases. Contract disputes, coverage decisions, utilization management programs, and formularies were all things that caused conflict between insurance companies, doctors and patients.

This laid a foundation for the thinking that insurance companies were only interested in profits, and willing to put patient care on the chopping block in the name of earnings. In some cases, though certainly not all, these indictments were true. No company is perfect, and the insurance companies are no exception. I worked for the insurance industry from 1987 through 2004 and know of many examples where insurance companies put profits ahead of what most people would consider good patient care. I can also tell you an almost equal number of stories where the insurance company was vilified just because it was an easy target and it really didn't do anything wrong.

The same holds true for the other actors in this play. I have seen good, honest doctors just as I have seen physicians who do things for monetary gain and not because it's clinically correct. Hospitals and employers all have the same positive and negative issues. The point is, in any system as big as healthcare, it's not so simple to figure out who is the hero and who is the villain. If there truly was a single "bad guy" to focus on, the problems would be much easier to solve.

That said, though, the expansion of the employer-based managed care system did produce some problematic side effects. The first was uncontrollable and unsustainable cost increases, the second was an increasing population of uninsured. Both of these factors were major players in the passing of the ACA. Put simply, if not for the hyperinflation of healthcare costs, and the 40 million-plus people in this country without insurance, there wouldn't even have been a debate on healthcare reform—let alone a bill and a vote in Congress. Because of this, it's important to address the issues of healthcare "hyperinflation" and the uninsured population separately, before we examine the current state of affairs in healthcare, and finally, what the future looks like.

CHAPTER 4

Healthcare Hyperinflation and the Uninsured

I n the truest sense, healthcare in this country is not hyperinflating by strict economic terms. However, given the amount of the U.S. economy devoted to healthcare and the impact that it can have on the world economy, even minor inflation can be staggering.

For more than 50 years, healthcare in America has had a steady track record of growing faster than the economy overall. This means that every year for the past five decades, healthcare has become a larger and larger part of the U.S. economy. Since this is a zero-sum game, the growth of healthcare means that other segments of the U.S. economy have had to shrink. This crowding out effect may or may not be good depending on your feelings about the industries or segments that were reduced. For example, in 1960, at 10% of GDP, the U. S. Department of Defense was twice the size of the healthcare market segment. In 2016, healthcare will account for around 17% of the U.S. economy while the Defense Department is down to 5%. Healthcare has more than tripled in the last 55 years while the Defense Department's portion of the U.S. economy has been cut in half.

Some people may view it as a positive that we're spending more money on healthcare and less on war while others, whose businesses may rely on defense spending, may view this as a negative. The problem is that industries other than defense have been crowded out by the increase in healthcare spending. In 1960, manufacturing accounted for 25% of the U.S. GDP. By 2015 that number had dropped to just 12%.

Healthcare is one of the big reasons the U.S. economy has been changing from a manufacturing and agricultural economy to a service-based one. This shift puts pressure on our economy as we purchase more and more durable goods from other countries, which fuels both trade deficits and federal budget deficits. So far, the U.S. economy has been able to withstand this shift from production, agriculture, and natural resource harvesting to a more service-based mix. The question from most economists is what happens when we reach the limit of that ability? What happens when the U.S. economy stops growing or even declines? What happens when unemployment goes up, along with interest rates and the national debt, and we don't have a production-based economy to fall back on? The last time the U.S. economy faced a significant downturn was the Great Depression, and we bounced back from that largely because we were still an agricultural and production-based economy. Now that we've seen those segments significantly erode, it may be more difficult to recover from future economic downturns.

What caused this inflationary trend, and how did it help create an environment ripe for the passage of the Affordable Care Act? Many factors led to inflationary pressures in healthcare. We have all listened to people talking about the ageing population, advances in technology, and innovation as factors driving up the cost of care. These all have an influence, but they really only tell part of the story.

Healthcare as an economic marketplace violates almost every rule that economists could set for an efficient market. In the eyes of an economist, healthcare in this country is set up for failure. While the problems with healthcare are many, three economic factors paint a clear picture of why it continues to become more expensive, and the changes that are going to be necessary to reverse this trend.

1. The purchaser is not the consumer. In any efficient economic market, it is critical that the consumer is also the purchaser. This means that the consumer is responsible for the results of his or her purchasing decisions. Every day as consumers, we weigh the consequences and make purchasing decisions. Going back to my car examples, on a regular basis people make purchasing decisions about automobiles based on their own set of criteria. One criterion is knowing that whatever amount of money they spend on a car will not be available to spend on other things. People calculate how much of a car payment they can afford and then shop for cars that fit that budget.

Imagine how those purchasing decisions would change if the consumer were insulated from the cost of his or her purchasing decisions. This is exactly how most healthcare is financed. In most cases the consumer (patient) is not the majority purchaser. The purchaser in healthcare is the employer or the government. Patients, in most cases, must pay only a small portion of the bill, thus insulating them from the effects of their purchasing decisions. This violation of Economics 101 is a significant factor in healthcare inflation.

Now, some people will argue that you can't compare healthcare and cars because people would still pay more for healthcare even if they *were* the purchaser; people won't put their health at risk. I think that argument lacks merit or evidence and use the development of the airbag in the auto industry as an example. Airbags were first developed in the early 1970s and were abandoned as an option on cars in 1977 due to lack of interest from consumers. Basically, consumers were not willing to spend the extra money for an option that could have a dramatic effect on their health and wellbeing. In 1984, the federal government had to pass legislation making passive restraints (air bags) mandatory in order for widespread adoption of this life-saving technology.

This and other examples that illustrate the consumer's willingness to trade health and wellbeing for money suggest that if the consumer of healthcare services were also the purchaser of those services, some very different purchasing decisions would be made. Economists and industry experts point out that if patients had to pay for their own healthcare they would do a great deal more "price shopping" than they do now, which could and would create a market dynamic that would drive down costs and help control inflation.

2. The supplier controls demand. The fundamental premise of economics is the law of supply and demand. We learn early on about supply and demand curves and how the interaction of the supply market, along with consumer demand, dictates prices. We also learn that things like cartels and monopolies that can control supply levels can manipulate prices and cause inflation.

What we don't focus on very much are markets where the supplier controls demand—which is the situation when it comes to healthcare. In most markets, the consumer decides what things they demand, how much they are willing to pay, and how much they want to buy. For example, when you go into a restaurant for dinner, you sit down and look over the menu. You decide what you are going to order and how much you are willing to spend. You may decide that you are in the mood for a nice steak and a salad. You would like a glass of wine and decide that a glass of the house red will do. And since you are already splurging on steak there will be no room in the evening budget for dessert.

This is a perfect example of consumers making purchasing decisions. No matter how much the waiter may try to sell you dessert, the final decision is yours. Now imagine that going out to eat was like going to the doctor. You sit down and the waiter comes by and asks you some questions about how hungry you are and what kinds of foods you like. You never see a menu or any prices. After hearing your answers, the waiter fills out your order. He tells you that you are going to have shrimp appetizer, steak, and salad. He orders an expensive bottle of wine and the baked Alaska for dessert. The bill is large but you don't care because first of all, someone else has to pay for it, and secondly, you didn't get to see the menu to determine if there was anything cheaper available.

Now I know patients must give permission for whatever treatment they ultimately receive. That said, we have all experienced a night out for a business dinner where the bill was on someone else's credit card and the host orders for the table. In those situations, have you ever seen anyone question the wine choice or argue that there were way too many appetizers for the table? If you go to your doctor with a headache and she frowns and suggests you should have some blood work, an eye exam, and an MRI, would you say no?

3. These are not rational decisions. The final problem with healthcare is the problem of rationale decision making. Economists talk about rational decision making as a key factor in establishing an efficient marketplace with market-based pricing. The problem with healthcare is it's not a rationale decision. No one ever shops for a cheaper surgeon who has a higher mortality rate. No one ever says, "Hey, do you have a cheaper chemo drug that isn't quite as good but doesn't cost so much." Trading cost for increases in risk is something we do every day in other purchasing decisions, but not something we as a society are comfortable doing in healthcare. This, too, serves to increase the inflationary predisposition of healthcare.

Combine these factors and you see why, and how, healthcare has had such a long run of staggering cost increases. Combine the factors we've discussed that lead to cost increases in healthcare with the structural flaws in its finance and delivery mechanisms and you get an environment where cost *control* is nearly impossible. Now, though, rather than ask "how did this happen?" we should be trying to determine what has to change to reverse this trend before it's too late. That question will be dealt with later in this book.

The next item that needs further discussion is the issue of the uninsured population in this country. Prior to the passage of the Affordable Care Act, everyone was talking about 47 million Americans who are uninsured. In several public addresses, the president even referred to the 47 million uninsured Americans who need help. Right up front, we need to recognize that there were *not* 47 million uninsured Americans nor have there ever been. That's right: the president gave you inaccurate information.

It's accurate to say that according to the latest census data there were 47 million uninsured people living in this country. However, roughly 10 million of those are not American citizens. Those 10 million people are undocumented immigrants living in this country. Now, it's an entirely different debate to address what, if any, obligation we *do* have for providing insurance to people in this country who are not citizens. The point is, if we're to subscribe to the belief that healthcare is a right of all Americans, and that it is our obligation to provide affordable health insurance for every citizen, then we need to begin with the more accurate pre-ACA number of 37 million uninsured Americans.

Once we accept our new pre-ACA starting point, we'll need to further dissect that number. Again, according to the most recent census, there are some interesting statistics about this population.

First, 60% of the uninsured population reported that they were in "excellent health." How many of these people could afford health insurance but are choosing not to buy it because they won't be using it? In addition, 16 million of the uninsured population reported a family income that is over $50,000 per year, which is higher than the mean family income in this country, and half of those 16 million reported making over $75,000 per year. I think it's fair to say that most, if not all, of this population could afford health insurance given their income levels.

Another interesting statistic is that 45% of the uninsured population was uninsured for fewer than four months. These are people who are uninsured for a very short period of time while they changed jobs or carriers. According to the Kaiser Foundation, the number of people who were uninsured for more than one year, did not qualify for Medicare or Medicaid, and made less than $50,000 per year numbered about 8 million. This represents about 3% of the population in this country.

Now that we better understand the population that was uninsured prior to the passage of the Affordable Care Act, we have a better point of reference to continue the discussion of the uninsured population in this country.

No matter the facts of the issue, the inflationary track record of healthcare over the past several decades, along with the belief that 47 million Americans were walking around with no healthcare and no ability to get healthcare, created a ripe environment for the development and passage of the Affordable Care Act. When you combine these factors with a period of time when one party controlled not only the White House but also the House of Representatives and the Senate, you have a political perfect storm.

Now you only need to understand the mind of the average elected official and his or her overriding desire to get re-elected and it all become perfectly clear. "You mean we could do something that could benefit somewhere between 20 and 40 million potential voters? Where do I sign!" I am reminded of the scene in the first "Ghostbusters" movie. Bill Murray's character is trying to get the mayor of New York to let him handle the ghost problem. He puts his arm around the mayor and says; "Lenny. Just think. You could be responsible for saving the lives of millions of registered voters." The mayor quickly decides that this would be a good thing.

Maybe I am being too critical of the motives of the people who wrote and passed the ACA. Then again, given this most recent election cycle, I have come to the conclusion that you can never underestimate the motives of an elected official.

With that background, let's move on to a hard look at the Affordable Care Act itself.

CHAPTER 5

The Affordable Care Act

As we have discussed, in 2010, President Barak Obama signed into law the Patient Protection and Affordable Care Act, or ACA. This was, without a doubt, the signature piece of legislation for his administration and the most sweeping piece of healthcare legislation since the creation of Medicare and Medicaid in 1965. Nancy Pelosi, the Speaker of the House when the bill was being debated, was almost prophetic when she said, "We have to pass the bill to find out what's in it."

In the beginning there was a great deal of debate as to what the new law would and wouldn't do. Several aspects of the law are only now becoming clear—more than five years later. To begin, let's examine the major parts of the law and what it was intended to do. After that, we'll need to examine how well the implementation of the ACA has worked and whether it met its goals. Finally, we need to evaluate the negative side effects of the law and how it's likely to shape the future of healthcare in this country.

The crafters of the ACA had a number of goals in mind when they put together the bill that eventually became law. In the beginning, they wanted to include a series of insurance reforms, incentives for individuals to buy health insurance, tax penalties for individuals who *didn't* buy insurance, and more tax penalties for businesses who didn't offer insurance to their employees. They also envisioned a national market place where anyone could purchase health insurance along with a new competitor in the market called the "public option." The public option was designed to be a government-run insurance plan.

The last major segment of the bill included an expansion of Medicaid to help more low-income individuals qualify for coverage under that program. The primary goals of the ACA were to reduce the number of uninsured people in this country, protect consumers from unsavory business practices of insurance companies, all while controlling the cost of healthcare.

There you have it: a one-paragraph summary of a piece of legislation more than 2,000 pages in the printing.

Too bad it's not that simple.

By the time it was enacted, most of what the Obama administration wanted made it into the law, with the notable exception of the public option. The public option was considered by its supporters to be a necessary part of the bill to keep the insurance companies honest. It was suggested that having a government competitor in the new healthcare marketplaces, which came to be known as "exchanges," was critical to the success of the plan. The problem was that the creation of a new government insurance company scared many people; it played directly into the hands of the Republican spin that government was going to "take over your healthcare." Late in 2009 the public option was deemed a bridge too far and threatened the bill's chance of passing the House of Representatives. A political decision was made to remove that provision and get the bill passed. That decision will turn out to be very important later as we examine the success or failure of the healthcare exchanges.

The public option may not have passed, but what did make it into law has already left a prominent, and likely lasting, impression on the healthcare landscape in America. To fully understand where healthcare is headed in the future you need to understand the basics of the Affordable Care Act and how it fundamentally changed healthcare in this country. Before we do that, it's useful to take a quick look at what many people feel was the precursor to healthcare reform and may have been the blueprint for the new law. We'll need to go all the way back to 1993, when Stanford economist Alain Enthoven wrote a paper called "Managed Competition." In his white paper, Enthoven outlined the steps necessary to fix healthcare inflation in this country. His prescription reads very much like what ended up in the ACA.

Enthoven called for the creation of uniform benefit plans so that consumers could effectively price shop carriers without trying to figure out the benefit differentials. The ACA created actuarially equivalent benefit plans in the form of the Bronze, Silver, Gold, and Platinum plans. Because these plans are actuarially equivalent, consumers can compare the offerings from different insurance companies on an apples-to-apples basis. While one carrier may have a higher co-pay but a lower deductible than their competitor, the consumer can be assured that if both plans are "Bronze" they will cover the same portion of total expected healthcare expenses, thus neutralizing any benefit differentials. Enthoven then called for forced universal coverage so that there were no "free riders" in the system. While the ACA didn't force universal coverage, the employer and individual mandates are clearly steps in that direction.

Enthoven wrote that an insurance marketplace needed to be created with transparent pricing. He went on to say that this marketplace would begin to create competition not only between health plans but also between delivery systems. Today we see the healthcare exchanges as the one market where transparent pricing is present. We also see competition not only between plans but also delivery systems, as tiered or sub-set networks are being developed around those delivery systems. The prices that follow those insurance products are reflective of the costs associated with the specific hospital system. In my area of Raleigh, North Carolina, we have the Duke University system and the University of North Carolina system operating very close to each other. We now see products built around those two systems that are competing with each other on the exchange.

What's most interesting is Enthoven's predicted end-game. Enthoven wrote that these changes in healthcare would drive budget-based capitation, which would end fee-for-service medicine and create a more efficient healthcare delivery system and marketplace. Under capitation, delivery systems or networks of providers are pre-paid a fixed amount to provide care to a given population of patients. Under this system, services like imaging become expenses to the delivery systems and not revenue generators. That profound change could turn the healthcare system in this country upside down.

While I agree with Enthoven that his could be the cure we've been looking for to our inflationary ills, we need to be cautious and mindful that many cures have significant side effects. It's like the old joke that the positive thing about a terminal illness is you never get it twice. More on this later.

So, knowing where the blueprint of the ACA came from, let's examine its major components and how they have already impacted healthcare in the United States.

1. The employer mandate. Part of the ACA was to create penalties for employers with over 50 employees who fail to provide healthcare coverage for their employees. The penalty for 2016 is $2,160 for each employee with the first 30 employees free. This is the part of the ACA that is designed to make sure larger employers offer coverage for their employees. The problems are that it does not affect small employers with fewer than 50 employees, and the penalty is much less than the actual cost of providing health insurance.

The significance of this should not be overlooked. The ACA, through its employer mandates and penalty levels, created a number of incentives in the labor market. First, since only full-time employees are counted, it creates an incentive for companies to have fewer full-time employees and more part-time employees. This is even more significant for those employers right around the 50-employee level. An employer who has 55 full-time employees but historically didn't provide insurance for those employees is faced with one of three options:

The first option is to provide insurance for their 55 employees at an average employer cost of $4,500 per employee. This means the employer just added almost $250,000 of expense to his or her business. The next option is to continue not covering the employees and pay the penalty. In this case the penalty would be 2,160 times 25 employees (remember you get the first 30 for free). So, instead of adding $250,000 of expense the penalty only adds $54,000 of expense to the budget. The final option would be to convert six employees to part-time and get down to 49 full-time employees. This means the employer pays no penalty at all. The negative impacts of this are that six employees lose their full-time employment and that this business now has a financial disincentive for growth.

You can see how some of the critics of the ACA refer to it as a job killer. While I haven't seen any good data to support the actual impact the ACA has had on unemployment, I think everyone would agree the incentives are still there for some businesses to either drop coverage and pay the penalty or convert to part-time employees to avoid the coverage requirement. Both of these are less-expensive options than paying for insurance for their employees. This impact is probably not widely felt in a good economy, where employers use benefits as a recruitment tool to help them secure labor. If the country ever experiences significant unemployment, though, and employers can attract and retain labor without offering benefits, we may see large employers drop coverage all over the country.

2. The individual mandate. The mirror image of the employer mandate is the individual mandate. Under the individual mandate, anyone who fails to purchase qualifying coverage pays a penalty. The penalty is 2.5% of the yearly household income that is above the minimum tax filing amount, or $695 per person. While this does create an incentive to purchase coverage, it's been argued that for many people, the penalty is much less expensive than purchasing insurance, even after government subsidies, and as such does not force the kind of universal coverage that Enthoven called for in his white paper about managed competition.

3. Medicaid expansion and Federal Subsidies. The ACA expanded coverage further by expanding the Medicaid program and offering federal subsidies for those individuals who didn't qualify for Medicaid up to a certain income level. The plan was for Medicaid coverage to be expanded to include individuals making up to 138% of the federal poverty level. Federal subsidies were provided to individuals to purchase insurance on the exchanges, paying for some or all of the cost of the coverage, with incomes up to 400% of the federal poverty level.

That was the plan, but the plan hit a snag at the U.S. Supreme Court. In 2012, part of the ruling on the case of *NIFB v. Seleblius* was to uphold the legality of the ACA, it was deemed not to violate the Commerce Clause because the penalty called for in the individual mandate was really a *tax* and was allowed under the Constitution. Further, the Supreme Court ruled that the federal government could not require that states expand Medicaid; this allowed states to opt out of this part of the ACA. To date, about half of the states have chosen to opt out of the Medicaid expansion program, limiting the law's impact on the uninsured population.

4. Healthcare Exchanges. The ACA created what I like to call "Travelocity for health insurance" with the state and federal healthcare exchanges. We now have a fairly simple marketplace where consumers can shop for insurance coverage of varying levels (Platinum, Gold, Silver, Bronze), offered by a number of insurance companies, some with different networks, and quickly see the cost difference for their choices. It's also a place where consumers can factor in any government subsidies and know what their monthly premium will be for various levels of coverage. They can make their selections and enroll right from the site. Sounds good so far right? Well, in many ways it is good. For many consumers, the exchange, combined with government subsidies, has provided them with an opportunity to purchase health insurance that they can afford for the very first time. However, like everything else, this development is not without its harmful side effects.

The creation of the healthcare exchanges fundamentally changed the way we purchase health insurance. I don't think it was fully understood by the drafters of the bill just how much that process would be altered, and it's only now becoming clear. Before the invention of the exchanges, most non-governmental health insurance was bought and sold at the employer level. This gave insurance companies some assurance that risk would be spread and predictable.

If an insurance company is bidding on an employer with 500 employees, covering a total of 1,200 people, they can be relatively assured that they will get a normal distribution of risk and cost. Of course, there will be individuals in the group with serious illnesses or conditions, but there will also be an offsetting population of young, healthy people to balance that cost. This is critically important in healthcare because costs are so concentrated. Remember, in the United States, half of all healthcare costs are spent on 5% of the population. By contrast 50% of the population only uses 3% of all the dollars spent on healthcare. The idea of getting a normal distribution is critical for health insurance. If a company gets too many of the most expensive 5% of the population, the numbers don't work. Inversely, if an insurance company can figure out how to get a greater portion of the 50% of the population who don't use healthcare, they can make a huge profit.

What does this have to do with the exchanges? Once the exchanges were created, the sale of insurance for that population went from employer-based, where one insurer would get the whole population of a given employer group, to individual purchasing. When you move to individual decisions, it changes the game completely. In the exchanges, the carriers must attract as many of the young, healthy people as possible while trying to avoid the older, sicker individuals. The insurance companies know that young, healthy people are price-shoppers and older, chronically ill people are more value and network shoppers.

To put it another way, a 58-year-old female who is battling multiple sclerosis, has been working with a sub-specialized neurologist for years, and is now on very expensive infusion therapy to handle her disease, is probably willing to pay a little more to make sure her neurologist and the place where she gets her infusions are in network. A 25-year-old healthy male doesn't care if there are any neurologists in the network and is likely to choose a plan based simply on price. So, if you are an insurance company, you need to enroll the 25-year-old male and would like to avoid the $50,000 a year drug costs that come with the 58-year-old MS patient. One way to do that is to drop the really good neurologist from your network. He will advise his patients to seek other insurance that includes his practice in their network. For every MS patient who switches from Insurance Company A to Insurance Company B, the medical expense, and therefor premium price, shifts from one to the other. This vicious cycle is called "adverse selection" and can cause Insurance Company B to also drop the neurologist in order to survive.

Think this couldn't happen? When BCBS of Minnesota rolled out their first Bronze plan on the new exchange, the network for that plan didn't include the Mayo Clinic. Many believe that this move was made for two reasons. One is that the Mayo Clinic is more expensive than other facilities in the area. However, many industry experts, including me, believe a stronger argument can be made for the other reason: to keep from attracting too many patients *of* the Mayo Clinic. If you need the Mayo Clinic, you're probably in that expensive top 5%. The insurance companies don't want you. It's probably also true that not many 25-year-olds chose someone other than BCBS simply because they couldn't get access to the Mayo Clinic.

An individual marketplace like the healthcare exchanges comes with some negative consequences. In this case, it creates an incentive for insurance companies to have a cheap network and avoid some of the very best specialists and facilities.

5. Insurance Reform. Probably the only part of the ACA that was widely agreed upon was the host of insurance reforms contained in the law. Insurance companies are almost universally hated, making it easy to get support for the idea of "sticking it to the big HMOs." From my perspective as a former managed care executive, I have to say I agree with most of the reforms in the ACA. Things like no life-time maximum and limited medical underwriting are long overdue.

That being said, I do think that the ACA went a bit too far with the new regulations, and this over reach may come back to haunt us in the future. The biggest problem I have with the insurance reform in the ACA is the medical loss ratio cap, or MLR. The MLR is the percentage of premium revenues that are paid for care delivery or quality improvement. So, if a plan has an 80% MLR, that means 80% of all premium revenues are paid out in claims payments; the remaining 20% is what the insurance company can use for administration, marketing, and profit. Under the ACA, plans *must* have an MRL of no less than 80% for the individual and small-group market and 85% for the large-group market.

Let's consider this for a moment without the bias against insurance companies. We now have a whole industry that is profit-regulated by the federal government. Say an insurance company does a great job of controlling costs. They collect $100 million in revenue, and because of their efforts at case management, preventative healthcare, and education, they have only $75 million in claims. Let's say their administrative costs for running the plan are $12 million. In most industries, that company would enjoy profits of $13 million, or a profit margin of 13%. Before you get all hot and bothered about $13 million in profits or a 13% margin, please keep in mind that Apple Corporation has a profit margin of almost 40% and I don't see anyone picketing their offices. Under the ACA, this plan would be forced to return between $5 million and $10 million dollars to its customers to meet the MLR requirements. This means their profit is capped at something in the neighborhood of 4% to 9%, depending on their mix of small-group to large-group business. This creates an environment where profits are limited but losses are not. It's a bit like going to Vegas and knowing you can lose money, but if you get lucky and hit a jackpot, the government is going to make you give back most of the money to the house.

It's true that the ACA also includes a number of protections for insurance companies. However, as we will see in the next chapter, most of these protections had a short life span. Even when they were in place, they fell woefully short of keeping the insurance companies from losing significant amounts of money in this new market place.

Now that we have a basic understanding of the ACA, what it was designed to do, and how it works, we can move on to examine the state of healthcare in this country today. It's time to examine the patient and fully embrace the good, the bad, and the ugly in our current environment. I'm going to warn you, things get a bit bumpy from here on out.

CHAPTER 6

Healthcare Today

At the time I'm writing this, we're six years into the Affordable Care Act, and the healthcare landscape is becoming more clear and, at the same time, more concerning. It is helpful to consider what has changed over the past six years as a way to get some early insight into what might be the successes and failures of the ACA. An evaluation of the condition of the market and its players will round out the information we need to make some predictions for the future of healthcare in this country.

Let's begin with the uninsured population. You will recall that before the ACA, we were counting roughly 47 million uninsured people in this country. That means that about 18% of the population of the United States didn't have coverage. One of the things we were promised the Affordable Care Act would do was reduce the number of people without insurance. While it's true that the number has come down, many would argue it hasn't come down enough, or as much as promised. Because of this, we still have a significant problem with the uninsured. The latest numbers show 11% of the population, 31 million people, still without insurance.

There is a long list of reasons why that number is still so high, but notably we have the Medicaid expansion being adopted by only a limited number of states, and the individual and employer mandates that don't have enough teeth to them to achieve their purpose. No matter the reason, we can safely conclude that unless further changes are made, the ACA alone will not solve the problem of the uninsured. Reality has fallen well short of the promises and projections made during the debate of the Affordable Care Act.

The fact that more than half of the pre-ACA uninsured remain so puts pressure on the system. Enthoven was correct when he pointed out that in order for the system to work, you had to force universal coverage. If there are a significant number of "free riders" it will undermine the whole situation.

The next thing to examine is cost control. The very name of the bill speaks to "affordable" care, so it's fair to ask if healthcare became more affordable over the past five years. The answer is again a bit mixed. In one sense, healthcare for millions of Americans *did* become more affordable. For those people purchasing insurance on the exchanges, and potentially receiving federal subsidies, healthcare became less expensive. However, when you look at it from a macroeconomic perspective, it's clear that the Affordable Care Act didn't do much of anything to reduce costs or control the inflationary trends from the past. The data would actually suggest the opposite, that the Affordable Care Act helped *accelerate* the rate of inflation in healthcare.

Let's look at two indicators: CPI-M and CPI-U. Healthcare inflation (CPI-M) is increasing faster than general inflation (CPI-U). When we look at the five-year period prior to the passage of the Affordable Care Act, we see CPI-M rose 1.5 times faster than CPI-U. When we look at the five-year period right after the passage of the Affordable Care Act, that number increased to 1.8 times faster than CPI-U. That would suggest that the passage of the ACA actually made matters *worse* in terms of the cost of medical care.

Now that we know the Affordable Care Act was only partially successful in eliminating the uninsured problem, and we know that it was not at all successful in controlling cost increases, we should move on to looking at the various players in the healthcare market to determine the winners and losers. In the current environment, we can look at physicians, hospitals, pharmaceutical companies, and insurance companies as the major actors. Understanding which of these players are currently winning and which are losing will help us understand how healthcare may evolve in the future and will tell us who is going to be resistant to change compared to who will welcome it.

PHYSICIANS

If there is a clear loser in the current environment, not to mention for the past couple of decades, it's physicians. From 1990 to 2013, physician salaries and incomes have actually lost ground to inflation. While the loss has not been sizeable, it's one of the only segments of the professional labor force that has experienced a decline in income when adjusted for inflation. There are also many reports of increased hours worked by physicians during this same time period. Working more and making less is not a recipe for success and is certainly not sustainable. I am concerned about how the physician market will react to any more bad news, or even a continuation of the status quo. The simple question is how much longer can physicians continue on this path? What makes this even worse is the fact that the entire healthcare sector has been growing so dramatically over the past 50 to 60 years. Physicians are one of the few major participants in the healthcare market to have "missed the party" financially.

HOSPITALS

The picture for hospitals is much better. While the data available on hospital profitability isn't great, since most hospitals aren't for-profit entities that are required to report results to the SEC, there is one measure that points to hospitals being winners in the current environment. If we take a time-lapse look at the portion of hospitals that have negative total or operating margins, we'll see when those hospitals' financial health improves or declines. In 1998, more than 40% of all hospitals had a negative operating margin and over 30% had a negative total margin. By 2014 those numbers had dropped by 10 points: only 30% of the hospitals had a negative operating margin and 20% had a negative total margin.

While we can't draw the conclusion that the ACA is the only reason for this improvement, it does seem logical that the ACA has helped hospitals more than it has helped physicians. Just think about the partial reduction of the uninsured and the impact that it has on hospitals. A reduction in the uninsured population means a reduction in the indigent care load on hospitals. Further, many of these people who obtained insurance for the first time had significant health issues that resulted in an increase in demand for hospital-based services, further driving profits.

The father of a friend of mine works with hospitals on the West Coast. He's told stories of patients coming in with minor complaints getting "every test on the menu" because now the patient has insurance and it'll get paid for. These patients aren't getting unnecessary care, but if it can be justified in any way, the hospitals are adding procedures to the tab. "People come in with a sprained ankle and leave with a new hip and two new knees!" is a joke probably not far from the truth in many cases.

INSURANCE COMPANIES

The other clear losers in the current environment are the insurance companies. This is probably the most surprising and unexpected result of the passage of the Affordable Care Act. During the debate prior to the passage of the bill, many individuals viewed the ACA as a huge win for insurance companies. Think about it: the government was going to make it easier for people to buy their product (federal subsidies and the exchanges), while at the same time enacting penalties for individuals who didn't get coverage, and for employers who didn't provide coverage (the individual and employer mandates). Can you imagine how happy the U.S. auto industry would be if the government announced a low-income subsidy for the purchase of an American-made car and a $3,000 penalty for anyone who didn't by a car if they didn't already own one? The stock price of the big three auto manufacturers would probably go up by 20% the day that law got passed!

The passage of the Affordable Care Act opened up the market to somewhere between 20 and 30 million potential new customers for insurance companies. Knowing nothing more than this, it's easy to see why many viewed this as a huge win for the health insurance industry. The problem is, health insurance is not a manufacturing industry like the auto industry is, and it's the differences that caused the problems. Looking back now, at the clues that were present then, it's easy to see that we had warning the insurance companies were not going to benefit from this new law.

The first clue was the reaction of Wall Street. Say what you will about Wall Street, but there are some pretty smart people working there whose sole job is to predict the future. They spend their lives trying to figure out if a company or industry is going to win or lose and do it before anyone else. Examined in that light, if the ACA were going to be an insurance company boon, we should have seen a jump in those companies' stock prices as an early reflection of their good fortune.

The fact is, Wall Street had the exact *opposite* reaction. If you look at the stock price of the five largest, publicly traded insurance companies (Aetna, Anthem, Cigna, Humana, and United) two years prior to the passage of the ACA (December 2007), and compare it to their prices right after the bill was signed into law (April 2010), you will see that Wall Street did not believe the payers were going to win. On the contrary, without exception, Wall Street predicted the insurance industry was going to be hurt by this new environment. Every one of those five companies saw a decrease in their stock price during that two-year period of at least 30%. The combined average decrease was more than 40%. What's even more alarming is if you look at the two-year period from 2005 to 2007, you see the average stock price change for these five companies is a 30% *increase* in value.

So, you have an industry where stock prices were rising by an average of 15% per year from 2005 to 2007 that from 2008 to 2010, as the Affordable Care Act gets debated, passed, and signed into law, saw an average decline in their stock price by over 20% per year. This should have been our first clue that the Affordable Care Act was going to be a problem, and that providing insurance under this new law was going to be very expensive and unprofitable for the carriers.

The second clue should have been the lukewarm reception given to the ACA exchanges by the national payers (Cigna, Aetna, Humana, and United). Rather than flock to a subsidized marketplace where a projected 20 million new customers could be found, the payers entered the market with great trepidation. Not a single national payer entered this market in every state, and in the states where they did offer their products, not a single one offered them in every county. Only the BCBS plans offered their products across the board, largely because of the significant political pressure that was put on each BCBS plan to do so.

The insurance companies now have two full years of ACA experience and the results are worse than anyone predicted, or could have even imagined. I wrote an article in 2013 titled "The ACA Death Spiral," where I predicted the demise of the exchanges and the mass exodus of payers from that market in 2017. When I wrote that article I assumed my predictions were a worst-case scenario. While it appears I got the timing right, as the national payers *are* leaving the exchanges in 2017, even my worst-case scenario as to the cost of this endeavor fell woefully short. Keep that in mind as you read further, especially as we get to my prediction of what the next five years might look like.

So the nationals have started leaving this market like rats jumping from a sinking ship. By the end of 2017 it's likely that if the national carriers participate at all in the exchanges it will be sparse at best. The more likely scenario is that the national carriers will be out completely by the end of 2017. That leaves only the BCBS plans and a few local insurance options to provide insurance for 12 million people.

The reason for this mass exodus is the simple fact that the cost of the people enrolling in the ACA exchanges is beyond anything that could have been predicted. The cost of that care is producing staggering losses. Some of the statistics are truly shocking. The national carriers all report significant losses with the limited experience they have had with the exchanges. Remember they cherry-picked the markets they entered and still they got stung. United HealthCare reports losses of over $1 billion in just two years. Aetna and Cigna report losses of close to $500 million each over two years.

Think about this for a moment. Three large insurance companies who make a living by estimating risk and pricing their products to that risk tiptoed into a new market, hand-picked the cities and states they believed would produce the best results, and in two years lost a combined $ 2 billion dollars. The BCBS experience has been no different. Every BCBS plan reports significant losses from the ACA. If you combine the financials for the nonprofit BCBS plans around the country, they posted a net *loss* in 2015. That hasn't happened in over 30 years. BCBS of North Carolina reports that the members they attracted in the exchange were 40% more costly than their average member before the ACA.

These losses and this experience have produced the beginning of the death spiral. The death spiral begins when a health insurance company starts losing money. The reaction is to raise premiums. However when you raise premiums, the young healthy people can no longer afford it and they drop out—which leaves you with an even sicker mix of people. That results in increased costs and more losses, which drives up premiums . . . thus the death spiral.

As we've already discussed, the fact of the matter is health insurance only works if you have enough young healthy people to make up for the small percentage of very sick people who use most of the services. We now know that the ACA exchanges have attracted some very expensive and sick people, and that the individual mandate and federal subsidies are not enough to attract, or force, enough young healthy people into the market to offset these costs. The result is the national companies have fled the scene and have left the various BCBS plans holding the proverbial bag. This development could have a significant negative impact on the delivery and financing of healthcare in this country beyond what anyone thought of when the law was passed. That will be explored later in this book.

BIG PHARMA

The only major winners in all of this seem to be the big pharmaceutical companies. The combination of Medicare Part D prescription benefits and the ACA adding 12 million covered lives—all with pharmacy benefits—has provided a serious boost to the profits of the pharmaceutical industry. In 2014, the biotech and pharmacy sectors worldwide produced revenues of over $1 trillion for the first time in history. To put that into perspective, if this industry were a country, it would be the 16th largest economy in the world just behind Mexico.

But massive revenues tell only part of the story. In 2014, the top 10 most profitable publicly traded healthcare companies were all in either the biotech or pharmaceutical industries. That's right, no insurance company stocks cracked the top 10. Seven of the 10 were biotech and the other three were pharma companies. Even more staggering are the profit margins these companies produce. Remember that the ACA, through the medical loss ratio requirement, effectively limited insurance companies to a profit margin of 3% to 4% on commercial insurance products. With that in mind, it's staggering that the top 10 most profitable biotech and pharmaceutical companies produced profit margins in 2014 ranging from 40% to 109%. Can you imagine being the CEO of a company that produces a 40% profit margin and being told by your board that you *failed* because nine of your peers did better?

While these are the 10 most profitable companies, the sector as a whole produced a profit margin of over 20%. So, if the ACA put the same kind of profit controls on pharmacy and biotech as it did on insurance, it would have reduced drug company profits—and therefore healthcare costs—by $160 billion in 2014 alone. I'm not suggesting the key to controlling costs is to enforce government profit controls in a free-market economy. Whenever that happens you have to look at the negative side effects. Just like raising the minimum wage leads to increases in unemployment, limiting corporate profits often results in a reduction in investment and innovation. The point of these statistics is to shed some light on the winners and losers in the healthcare environment today rather than prescribe solutions. The solutions will come a bit later.

As we look at the healthcare landscape today, we see a market that is inflating faster than overall economic growth can accommodate. We find a market that is massive and consuming an ever-increasing portion of the U.S. economy. We see a market that is negatively affecting not only governmental spending, but also the private sector. We see a market where there are few winners other than the big biotech and pharmaceutical companies and several significant losers. We see a market where the problem of the uninsured still hasn't been solved. Lastly our most recent solution, the Affordable Care Act, has not only failed to solve the problem of runaway inflation, but by all accounts, made it worse.

Simply put, we see a market that is poised for correction if we are lucky and collapse if we aren't. We see the economic version of the perfect storm. Hold on to your hats ladies and gentlemen it's going to get a little windy.

CHAPTER 7

Rationing

Now comes the part of the book that makes everyone cringe and want to skip to the next chapter. Please don't do that because this is a very difficult but important part of what we must discuss in order to truly deal with healthcare in this country. That's right, it's time to talk about rationing. See, you made a little face and got uncomfortable, didn't you? This is the problem with discussing rationing: it makes everyone uncomfortable. Be that as it may, we still have to have this discussion.

Let's start with some fundamental facts. These will help us navigate these difficult waters without losing our bearings—or humanity.

Every country in the world rations healthcare in some way, shape, or form. Some countries ration it through access. Some countries ration it through quality, or lack thereof, while others ration through income. For years, people have compared the U.S. healthcare system to the systems in Canada or Great Britain. The Canadian and English systems ration care mainly through access. Virtually everyone has *coverage* through the government; what they don't have is ready *access*. If you need a service, you are put on a waiting list. For many things, that list is short and you get care right away. For other things, you may wait a while before you get care.

For example, a study by the Commonwealth Fund reported that for non-life-threatening elective surgeries 33% of Canadians reported waiting more than four months while only 8% of Americans had to wait more than four months for the same type of service. Another study by the Frazier Institute reported that Canadians waited on average of more than 18 weeks from the time they saw a general practitioner to the time they received the necessary surgery or treatment for their condition. Both Canada and Great Britian are rationing care, they are just doing it in different ways. You may argue that rationing through access is better than what we do in this country and I wouldn't completely disagree with you. What you can't argue is that there is a way to provide healthcare without choosing some kind of rationing. That argument just doesn't hold water.

Another important fact to accept is that we ration almost everything in this country. We ration food, housing—almost anything you can think of that's purchased on the economy. That doesn't mean we withhold food or housing, but rather not everyone gets the same as everyone else. Not everyone has a house or lives in a great apartment. Not everyone has the same access to food. I'm not saying this is right or wrong, that's a whole different discussion for a different book not to be written by me. What I am saying is that rationing is a fact of life and, as such, something we should talk about when it comes to healthcare.

The reality is that we simply can't afford to provide everything to everyone. Anyone who says otherwise either doesn't understand what he or she is saying or is outright lying. If we've proven anything over the past 50 or 60 years, it's that trying to provide only the very best care, with incredible access, on the cutting edge of technology and advancement, will break the bank. It'll result in a significant number of our low-income citizens left with either limited or no access to that care. What we have proven over the past five years is that trying to create an artificial market to expand this kind of coverage to the millions of people left on the side of the healthcare roadway, while noble, will only make the problem worse.

Finally, what I believe we have done is ignore the primary impediment to controlling healthcare costs in this country. We've completely sidestepped the issue of how we are going to ration care so that we provide the most good for the most people without destroying our economy.

Consider the situation with organ transplants. As a society, we understand that there are a limited number of organs that can be used for transplants. We also understand that many times the demand for organs is greater than the supply, and because of this, people sometimes die while waiting for a transplant. To mitigate deaths as much as possible, we have developed a system that will prioritize the people on the transplant waiting list such that the limited supply of organs is utilized in a manner that has the best chance of long-term survival and success.

We also have come to terms with the fact that lifestyle choices and behaviors can get you removed from the list. Case in point: if you are waiting for a liver transplant you can't be an active alcoholic and expect to get an organ. This whole approach to transplants is a form of rationing and a very effective and logical one at that.

So what is the difference between accepting that there is a limited supply of organs and accepting that there is a limited supply of money? The answer is in the question. We haven't yet accepted that there is a limited supply of money, and our demand for healthcare exceeds that supply of money, and therefore our ability to pay for it. To me, this is the fundamental hurdle we face, and until we realize the truth and figure out the best way to ration our healthcare dollars, we are never going to fix the problem.

The last thing to keep in mind when thinking about rationing is this: rationing is nothing more than artificially dealing with a disconnect between demand and supply. Failure to do so will result in market forces doing it on their own. Eventually markets find a balance and the healthcare market is no different. The question isn't if this problem will ultimately get "fixed." Rather, the question we should be asking ourselves is whether would we rather deal with it in a logical fashion, as we have done with transplants, or let the market have its way. It's a bit like the old saying "All planes land eventually." While that's true, there's a big difference between a plane that lands safely, guided by a skilled pilot, and one that falls out of the sky. They both "landed," but I think you'll agree the ride down would be very different depending on which plane you were on.

CHAPTER 8

Healthcare for the Next Five Years

E veryone has heard the term "the widow maker." This is a massive heart attack that kills instantly and makes some poor woman a widow. You probably know someone or have heard of someone who had such a heart attack or got lucky and was told by a doctor that if they hadn't caught something they were likely to have one in the future. The title of this book suggests that healthcare could be that kind of heart attack for the U.S. economy. The title is not just marketing hype. I truly believe that if we don't do something soon, our economy could be at risk for a widow-maker event the likes of which we haven't seen since the Great Depression.

To be honest, I think a healthcare implosion could actually be worse than the Great Depression, because unlike the situation in 1929, the U.S. government today may not be able to spend its way out of an economic crisis. In 1929, the national debt was less than 20% of our country's GDP. By 1939, that number had gone up to about 44% of GDP. Think of it like this: In 1929, our country was carrying very little credit card debt. We had a problem and lost our job, so we lived on our credit cards until we could find work again. That only works if you have room on your credit card like we did in 1929.

Fast-forward to today. Today the federal debt is over 100% of GDP. That's right, we have more credit card debt than we do income, so to speak. Think about your own income level and how dangerous it would be to have more credit card debt than you make every year. Well ladies and gentlemen, that's the good old U.S. of A today. So, if we lose our job again we may find it hard to get anyone to increase our credit card limit. When a government is not able to borrow money to finance its deficits, the only option left is to print more currency. The problem with printing more money is it rapidly devalues the currency, which causes hyperinflation, which can become a vicious cycle. In post-World War I Germany, the world saw what hyperinflation could do. In 1921, it took 90 Deutsche marks to buy 1 U.S. dollar. By 1923, just two years later, each U.S. dollar was worth 4.2 *trillion* DM. That's not a typo. A U.S. dollar was worth 4.2 trillion marks. That's hyperinflation.

This chapter is devoted to painting a picture of what could happen if we don't address the issues facing the healthcare market. Let me begin by saying that this is not so much a prediction as it is an illustration of how the market may correct itself if we don't intervene. I also want to acknowledge up front that this is probably a worst-case scenario and should be viewed as such. That being said, while reading this chapter, you should keep asking yourself: "Could this really happen?" If you keep an open mind, your conclusion will be that it *absolutely* could happen. That's the scary part. So, with that understanding, let's look forward to the next several years and watch the collapse of the American healthcare system and the impact it would have on the U.S. economy.

2017

A new Republican administration and Republican-controlled Congress begin taking apart the Affordable Care Act and replacing those parts with their own ideas.

1. The new administration eliminates the individual and employer mandates in the ACA.
2. Federal funding for Medicaid expansion is rolled back, leaving the states to decide if they want to continue to fund the Medicaid expansion on their own.

3. Most of the states with Medicaid expansion realize they can't afford it without federal funding and return to previous Medicaid qualification levels.
4. The administration passes a series of tax cuts and deductions for individuals and businesses to help finance healthcare expenses, including premium payments.
5. The administration passes legislation designed to increase the usage of HSAs (Health Savings Accounts).
6. The final piece of legislation passed by the new Congress is a law that allows for the selling of health insurance across state lines.

These changes set the stage for the downfall of the healthcare exchanges and the early stages of a meltdown of the healthcare system in this country. The removal of the individual and employer mandates makes the insurance companies concerned that adverse selection in the exchanges will increase and the risk pool will get worse. Since the payers left in the exchanges are already losing significant money, the changes in 2017 will ultimately bring about the end of the ACA exchanges. Rolling back Medicaid expansion will take close to 10 million people and put them back onto the rolls of the uninsured. That moves the uninsured number up from its low point of about 17 million to around 27 million.

With the Republican win in the 2016 elections it is clear to me that major parts of the Affordable Care Act will be dismantled. I would expect the individual and employer mandates to be removed during the first few months of the new Congress. I certainly think we should expect the reinsurance pool *not* to be funded any further. These changes will have a dramatic impact on the BCBS plans and the few remaining regional insurance companies that still offer products on the ACA exchanges. The payers will conclude that the exchanges are never going to be profitable places to do business. They'll also know that with a Republican-controlled administration and Congress, leaving the exchanges will produce no governmental backlash. This will not only allow further exodus from the exchanges, but might actually push the payers in that direction.

2018

Healthcare costs continue to rise, the uninsured population increases, and payers make a mass exit of the ACA exchanges. This all sets the stage for further healthcare inflation, financial problems for providers, and increased budgetary concerns for state and federal governments.

1. Many of the BCBS plans across the country pull out of the exchanges, either totally or in major parts of each state, due to a deteriorating risk pool and continued financial losses. Combined with the previous exits of the national payers, this shows the current structure of the ACA and its healthcare exchanges is not sustainable without major overhaul.

2. With the exit of the plans from the exchanges, the uninsured population goes back up to pre-ACA levels, around 40 million. This puts financial pressure back on hospitals and physicians who are faced with providing care to patients who have no ability to pay. Hospitals and physicians in a position to demand higher rates from insurance companies do just that, which helps drive up the cost of insurance further. Those that don't have a dominant position begin to have financial difficulties.

3. Employers facing escalating healthcare costs and no employer mandate start scaling back coverage levels, and in many cases, drop coverage altogether. This puts further pressure on individual disposable income, which negatively affects the U.S. economy.

4. Medical CPI continues to track at rates close to twice general inflation, which continues to increase the portion of GDP consumed by healthcare. This begins to crowd out other economic activities like manufacturing.

2019

The country is back to an uninsured population of over 40 million and rising. Healthcare costs continue to inflate too rapidly and the impact on the U.S. economy begins to become problematic. The system is in the beginnings of a death spiral that may not be recoverable.

1. Medical expense increases along with the burden of the uninsured begin to have an impact on unemployment. Unemployment in 2019 rises to 6.5%. Economists grow concerned that this uptick in unemployment is the first time the country has seen such a trend since the housing crash of 2008.

2. The increase in unemployment along with the slowing of economic growth increases the federal deficit to $950 billion in 2019. The national debt is now above $20 trillion and is approaching the highest ratio of debt-to-GDP in U.S. history. The previous high was 119% in 1946 right after World War II. Economists predict that we could top 120% of GDP as early as 2022.

3. Interest rates begin to go up as China and other nations begin demanding higher returns on the purchase of U.S. debt due to concerns over the U.S. economy.

2020

The country is now in a full recession, with many signaling the possibility of a depression. Healthcare has caused a domino effect on several parts of the economy, resulting in a large-scale correction.

1. With economic growth all but stopped, unemployment levels go up to 10%. This is a level not seen since the housing crisis of 2008.

2. Interest rates start to spike, putting pressure on the U.S. economy and causing issues with the federal budget.

3. Healthcare providers start to feel the pinch. Many hospitals begin laying off staff. Drug companies begin layoffs to try and maintain profit levels. Physician groups begin limiting their Medicare and

Medicaid patients and many drop from one or both programs to provide care to patients with better reimbursement. Patients begin to complain about care and service in the hospital and many Medicare and Medicaid patients have difficulty finding doctors. This causes an influx of patients seeking non-emergency care in hospital ERs, which drives up costs and hinders the ability of those hospitals to provide emergency care in that setting.

4. The combination of increasing unemployment and increasing interest rates is a compounding problem for the federal budget. The deficit exceeds $1.4 trillion, which is almost 50% of the total tax revenue received. For the first time, the U.S. government is now spending 50% more than it collects in tax revenue.

5. Many economists begin warning that all indications point to a further decline in the economy, and that the country may be headed into territory that it hasn't seen since the Great Depression.

Ok, I'm going to stop here because to be honest, this is starting to make it hard for me to sleep at night. The end to this story should be apparent. Hospitals and physician groups start to fail and people can't get the care they need. Unemployment goes up as hospitals, physicians, and other related healthcare businesses lay people off in an attempt to stay afloat. Healthcare costs destroy the federal budget, which drives up deficits. Interest rates go up, which drives up deficits even further. Basically we enter the modern-day equivalent of the Great Depression.

As I stated at the beginning of this chapter, I am not predicting that all of this is going to happen. Rather, I'm trying to show what could happen, an illustration of how bad things could get. The questions for the reader are these: Are any of the predicted scenarios *not* possible? If most or all of them *are* at least possible, then what is the probability that some or all of them could happen if we don't do something to prevent them?

There is a great quote in the book and movie "The Big Short." *"People hate to think about bad things happening so they always underestimate their likelihood."*

With that said, I am going to take a moment, pour myself a stiff drink, and proceed to the next chapter of this book—trying to prescribe a cure that will help us avoid all of this. Wish me luck.

CHAPTER 9

The Prescription for the Cure

The prognosis for the healthcare system in this country isn't very good, and we have some serious issues that must be addressed. Adopting a "do nothing" or "watchful waiting" approach isn't going to work. The current environment is simply not sustainable. The Affordable Care Act didn't fix our problems and may even have made things worse. If we're going to avoid the coming collapse, something must actually be *done*. If you disagree with these statements please put my book down and pick up something else, fiction probably, because the first step to solving this problem is honestly admitting we *have* a problem. If you're not ready to do that, enjoy the latest book about teen vampires in love and leave the hard work of fixing this problem to the rest of us.

Now that they're gone, let's start talking about the cure.

Let's begin with the understanding that there is no magic pill for this one. There is no simple answer to a very complicated problem. There is no single villain for us to thwart. We're going to have to come to terms with the fact that the cure isn't going to be instant or painless. We are facing a problem that is decades in the making and has become life threatening—both figuratively and literally.

The first painful fact to acknowledge is we simply can't provide everything for everyone. Let's stop there and really let that sink in, because that may be the most important, most fundamental point. We are not going to be able to provide everything for everyone. I think any discussion of a cure for these problems begins and ends with a discussion of rationing healthcare in some way. You don't have to *like* that reality, but if you're going to develop a cure for our healthcare system, you do have to *accept* it.

I was speaking to a group of oncologists and others involved with cancer care a while back. After my presentation, the discussion moved to the issue of high-cost cancer treatments and why payers deny them or make it difficult to get them approved. We started talking about how to balance the amount of clinical benefit with the cost increase of a new therapy or treatment. The question I posed was this, "What would you do if a new drug came out that increased life expectancy by six months and only cost $10 more than the current drug you use?" The instant answer was obvious and unanimous; they all said they would start using the new drug on their patients. I then asked this, "Ok, what if that same six-month increase in life expectancy came at a cost of $100,000? Or $1 million for that matter?" It was a tougher question to answer, uncomfortable, but most—nearly all—of the people in that room agreed that they couldn't justify using a new $1 million drug to buy their patients six months of life.

In the conversation that followed, their responses to the drug question allowed me to take the position that we had just agreed life is not priceless, that it does have a monetary value. While we may disagree on how much should be spent for every extra month of life, we did agree that there is a limit to what we can spend in good conscience. If we could accept that position, we could move on to figuring out where the limit is, and from *there* we could have an honest discussion on how to do the most good for the most people given the fact that money is a limited resource.

The looks on the faces of the people in the crowd ranged from depressed to enlightened. They mostly were physicians who had dedicated their lives to doing the very best for their patients—typically regardless of the cost. While that's both a noble and honorable endeavor, there are economic consequences of that approach. Being suddenly confronted with the financial realities of our situation didn't sit well with many of them. One physician raised her hand and said, "Are you saying that I may have provided my best care yesterday and it's all downhill from here?" I responded by saying, "Yes and no. You may have provided your best care yesterday for *some* of the people who needed it. What I am saying is we need to move from a system that provides the very best care for some, to one that provides great care for *most*, or even very good care for *all.*"

Let's explore the idea of rationing and how we can employ it effectively.

Probably the most critical part of any solution to our healthcare woes is to figure out a way to ration care. Any time someone starts this discussion, very powerful emotions quickly boil to the surface. Images of people being left to die while life-saving care is available spring to our minds. We think of drugs being withheld solely because of price. We imagine surgeries not performed because some insurance executive or government official decided the patient was just too old to benefit from it. These and worse all come to the forefront.

I agree that these ideas are disturbing and should be avoided if we possibly can. I ask you to consider, though, how much worse is life in those images than the one we already have in this country? We have people taking half their necessary medication so they can afford food. Large segments of our population receive care in clinics that most of us would find unacceptable. Elderly patients are going without necessary care because they can't find a physician willing to see new Medicare patients. Are these situations really that much better?

Right now, we provide incredible care to many people, great care to most, and at least some care to all. This is the situation that is going to break the bank and leave us with only a few people able to afford healthcare and everyone else going without. Our mission when considering rationing is not to choose who gets their care covered and stop there, but to determine how to provide the best care we can to the most people without breaking the bank. How do we ration the financing of care so that the most people possible have paid access to it? Dealing honestly with the distasteful thoughts that rationing usually inspires is going to be integral to moving forward. Let's start with a focused approach to the use of rationing.

WHAT GETS COVERED

The first thing we need to address is a more logical and cost-effective way of deciding what gets covered. Every doctor I have ever met has a frustrating story about a service or drug being covered by one insurance company but not another. They tell of services covered by Medicare that commercial insurance companies *don't* pay for. They've been forced to jump through different hoops for different insurance companies just to get the *same service* covered for their patients. This process is confusing, illogical, and costly.

Think about it for a moment: the care you receive and the services or medications that are available to you are dependent on the insurance company you have—or maybe how skilled your physician is at filling out forms. Why should one patient get one level of care while a patient with the same condition doesn't get it just because of the insurance he or she has?

Let me give you a very real example. A lab company hired me to help them get their new lab test covered by more insurance companies. They had developed a single test that they believed did a better job measuring cardiac risk than the standard cholesterol tests. From the data I saw, they believed they were correct. The test they'd developed produced a more accurate measure of cardiac risk because it counted actual particles in the bloodstream rather than making an inference to the number based on the patient's total cholesterol score. The lab's medical director, a very good lipidemiologist, made a compelling case that if something is worth measuring it's worth measuring accurately, and their test was a more accurate measure of cardiac risk. He went on to point out that since the standard cholesterol test could either overstate or understate the number of particles, and because people have different amounts of cholesterol per particle, having a more accurate measure would help doctors correctly treat and control high cholesterol. He believed this would lead to fewer cardiac events.

All of this sounds good, right? The lab even had historic claims data from an expansive payer database that *proved* patients who had this test had fewer cardiac events than patients who were only managed with the standard test.

At the time I was brought in, the company's test was Medicare approved, but was only covered by about half the BCBS plans in the country. United HealthCare did approve the test and covered it; Cigna and Aetna did not approve the test at all. You're probably asking yourself, why would some BCBS plans, Cigna, and Aetna not approve a test that was clinically better and reduced cardiac events?

I have intentionally left two critical pieces of information out of the story. The first bit of information is the test was more than *twice* as expensive as any other test of its type. The second piece of information is that while the claims data showed the test did reduce cardiac events, the cost savings didn't cover the increased cost of the test itself. So, using the test, while clinically better, produced a higher total cost of care. In this example, people who had Medicare, or one of the health plans that covered this test, could get it. People who had one of the plans that didn't cover the test would have to pay for it themselves or decline the more advanced screening. Theoretically, there are probably people who ended up having a cardiac event because their doctor couldn't get them this test and therefore couldn't manage their cholesterol as well as he could the patients who did receive this test.

Before everyone starts ranting, let me clearly state: I am not qualified to determine if this particular test should or shouldn't be covered.

Both sides of this issue present good and compelling arguments. The point I'm making is that in the current environment, we have a disparity of coverage policies driven only by payer selection, and that produces problems of equity while also driving up costs. There must be a better way, and we'll get to it after we tackle something a little less emotionally charged: administrative waste.

Adding to the injury of inequity, we have the insult of waste and the administrative cost that comes with it. Every physician group has a person, or in the case of medium or large groups, a team, of people who do nothing but get authorizations for the services they want to provide. Each of these people/groups has a counterpart at the payers whose job it is to review these requests and approve or deny them. Every day hundreds of thousands, maybe *millions* of requests for authorization or pre-certification are sent from providers to payers to be reviewed and approved, denied or returned with a request for additional information. None of this activity is necessary for the actual provision of care, but it consumes precious healthcare dollars.

What if there was a way to eliminate all of this nonsense, create a single source for coverage policies, and reduce costs all at the same time? Wouldn't that be a good step toward fixing the problems we face? Of course it would, and here's how I think we do it:

The Omnibus Budget Reconciliation Act of 1989 created, among other things, the Relative Value Update Committee, also known as the RUC. The RUC is a committee of 31 people, 21 of whom are selected representatives from the national medical specialty societies. This committee makes recommendations to CMS on RVU changes and RVU assignments for new CPT Codes.

My suggestion is to broaden the committee's role to help us combat the problem we just discussed. The RUC could be tasked with developing and maintaining a set of national coverage policies and criteria. These policies and criteria would take into account not only clinical value but also the cost effectiveness of treatment options, new drugs, procedures, etcetera. The committee would also be tasked with setting recommended care pathways. These coverage policies and clinical pathways would be enforced for all payers, governmental and commercial. This would of course require a change to the current federal Medicare legislation, as well as the federal ERISA (Employee Retirement Income Security Act) legislation that governs self-funded plans, not to mention the Affordable Care Act, to cover fully insured plans. State Medicaid could be handled by tying federal funds to the adoption at a state level for the state Medicaid population.

These coverage policies should cover the vast majority of care delivery situations and patients. Understanding that no set of policies is going to cover 100% of the patients or situations, we'd need to retain existing appeal mechanisms to handle exceptions. This way, if patients or their physicians felt there was a strong argument to be made for an approach that differed from the national policy, they could appeal for an exception and have it paid for. These mechanisms are already in place for all governmental and private payer situations.

Further, these policies would be considered a minimum level of coverage. No plan could deny a treatment that followed the national policy. If, however, a self-funded employer wanted to provide additional coverage, they could do so, since they are fully responsible for the cost. If a commercial insurance company wanted to offer a plan with expanded coverage beyond the national set of policies, they could do that as well. The coverage policies would be designed to limit those services that could be denied and remove most, hopefully all, of the pre-certification and prior-authorization process.

The RUC's role would not be to simply slash the list of services that could be covered. For example, the national coverage policy would most likely be that medical treatment for infertility would not be required to be covered. Procedures like IVF would not be considered medically necessary and therefor the RUC would not require them to be paid for by insurance. However, if a self-funded employer *wanted* to provide that benefit for their employees, they could. A commercial insurance company may want to sell an "Infertility Rider" to those employer groups who wanted to purchase it. Each of these situations would be allowed.

Let's say the national coverage policy *did* cover services related to the diagnosis of infertility. In that case, no insurance company could deny the testing or other services necessary to diagnose infertility, nor could they require any pre-certification for these services. The process would be streamlined and at least some of the cost related to the treatment would be reduced.

Speaking of prior-authorization and pre-certification, an article in *Medical Economics Magazine* in 2014 referenced a 2011 study in *Health Affairs* that calculated the total cost of the prior-authorization process to physicians in this country at $69 billion dollars per year. If the payers who have to review and decide on all of these requests pay a similar cost, then eliminating the process saves almost $140 billion per year. To put that into perspective, in 2015, the federal government spent $69 billion on Medicare physician payments. By eliminating the administrative expense of prior-authorization, we could potentially save twice as much money as the federal government currently spends on Medicare payments to physicians. While this doesn't solve our whole problem, you know what they say: a billion here and a billion there eventually adds up to real money.

In addition to setting the policies for what will be covered, the RUC could set policies for when and under what conditions specific care would be covered. This gets us to heart of how we employ rationing. For example, a brain MRI obviously is something that should be covered. The question is, under what circumstances? A patient with a mild headache and no other symptoms or presentations should probably not be approved for an MRI. A patient with a severe headache and other presentations and symptoms that could indicate a tumor *would* be covered for an MRI. Again, appeal and exception processes would need to continue to account for unusual situations.

In order for this to work, the committee would need to have a mechanism not only for evaluating the clinical effectiveness of a treatment or drug, but also the economic impact of these coverage decisions. I propose that any and all policy coverage decisions or clinical pathways would be evaluated by the actuarial department of CMS to determine the cost or savings they would generate. The agreement would be that for any policy or pathway that was adopted, the Medicare conversion factor would be adjusted as a result of the added cost—or the generated savings—to federal healthcare spending.

Say that at the monthly RUC meeting several policies and pathways were adopted or adjusted. The net impact of these was a cost increase to Medicare. That cost increase would be offset by a reduction in the Medicare conversion factor for physicians as well as reductions in reimbursements to hospitals for Part A services. Conversely, if the adopted policies and pathways produced cost savings, the conversion factor and hospital payments would automatically increase. This zero-sum game would provide incentive for the RUC to be intelligent on what they approve or adopt because the physicians and specialties they represent would face the economic impacts of their decisions.

Let's take my previous example of the advanced cholesterol lab test and run it through this scenario. The company that developed the test would present it to the RUC for consideration. The RUC would review the relative clinical data and provide guidance to the CMS actuarial team for an economic analysis.

What if the RUC agrees that the test is better than the standard cholesterol test, but doesn't think it should be used for front-line screening due to its cost? They would develop a clinical pathway that identifies higher-risk patients they believe *would* benefit from this advanced test. They share that pathway with the CMS and the actuaries come back and say the adoption of the policy along with the clinical pathway would be cost neutral. The RUC then adopts the coverage policy along with the clinical pathway for which patients and circumstances will allow the test to be covered. We'd have the whole country getting access to a new test—but only where appropriate.

Let's take another more interesting scenario, one that demonstrates the way a national coverage policy could fundamentally change the way new drugs are introduced and priced in this country.

Drugs account for almost 10% of all healthcare costs, and in 2014, the overall price of drugs increased by more than 12% compared to the previous year. Pharmaceuticals account for a large portion of healthcare costs and have been inflating at a rapid pace. Keep in mind, too, that the current system really doesn't provide any incentive for drug companies to develop cheaper drugs. Rather, there is an incentive to focus solely on the development of drugs that are clinically better, because if they do, drug companies can charge almost whatever they want for them!

A perfect example is the drug Solvaldi for Hepatitis C, which hit the market in 2014 with a price tag of $1,000 per pill. Medicare alone spent $3.1 billion in 2014 on that *one drug.* I wonder if the drug would have been approved in my RUC scenario? With those things in mind consider the following:

A drug company develops a new drug that is almost as good as Solvaldi for Hep C patients. They show that for 95% of the patients, their new drug is just as good as Solvaldi. They price the drug at $500 per pill. The company presents their new drug to the RUC. The RUC agrees with the clinical findings and has CMS evaluate a policy adoption along with the pathway that identifies the 5% of the people who really need Solvaldi and allows them to continue with their medication as prescribed. CMS comes back with a savings of $1.475 billion and the coverage policy and pathway is approved. In one meeting, the manufacturer of Solvaldi loses $1.475 billion in Medicare revenue along with 95% of their non-Medicare Solvaldi revenue because of the policies set by the RUC.

What do you think the manufacturer is going to do? I think they're likely to approach the RUC with Solvaldi again, only this time with a price tag *not* set at $1,000 a pill but rather $400 per pill. This is quickly adopted by the RUC and we get another $275 million in savings. What we'd have is an efficient marketplace where price drives consumption. We'd have something that acts more like a free-market economy, which is very effective at controlling unnecessary inflation. The entire pharmacy industry, along with others, would now focus on producing more cost-effective and less-expensive drugs because they know that will drive market share.

Just think about how much this could impact overall healthcare expense. If this item alone produced a 10% reduction in pharmacy costs, it would drop total healthcare expenditures by 1% all by itself. We're on a roll, so let's move to the next way a form of rationing can help solve our problem.

END-OF-LIFE

We need to talk about end-of-life issues. Start with the facts: About 80% of the people who die every year are covered by Medicare. About 25% of the total money spent by Medicare each year is spent in the last year of someone's life. That means Medicare spends over $150 billion every year paying for the last year of life. If we do the math using 2014 as our basis, the average amount spent by Medicare per beneficiary in the last year of life was $34,539. That's four times the average cost of the same year for the remaining beneficiaries.

It's interesting to note the cost of a Medicare recipient's final year does not continue to increase with the age of the patient beyond a certain point. The peak cost happens at age 73 and then declines from there. This suggests that as a society, we get more comfortable with death as the patient gets older, more often choosing palliative care over more expensive and invasive services.

Before anyone gets upset, I am not suggesting that we withhold care for seniors. What I am suggesting is that there may be a better way to handle end-of-life care and decisions. In our current environment, we put families and physicians in a terrible position. We ask family members to make decisions about their loved ones that they are not equipped to make at a time when they're not in a good position emotionally to make them. We put physicians in the role of trying to advise family members without sounding callous or uncaring. The whole situation is set up to produce the kind of wasteful spending that needs to be addressed.

I would like to share a personal story that illustrates my point. Stories like this play out every day in hospitals and other facilities across the country.

My grandfather spent the last year of his life in a skilled nursing facility. He had lost his leg below the knee to diabetes and had lost a lot of weight. He suffered from dementia and most of the time thought he lived on his farm with the team of draft horses he had many years before. I was visiting him one day with my father when a very nice young man came in and started doing some measurements on my grandfather's stump. When I asked him what he was doing he said, "I'm fitting him for his prosthetic." I couldn't believe my ears. Here was an old man who weighed less than 90 pounds and was obviously nearing the end of his life. He was so weak I didn't think he could have walked with *four* good legs. When I asked the nurse why he was getting fitted for a prosthetic, his reply was; "Don't worry, Medicare will cover it."

At this point I started getting angry. "That's not my question. My question is why are you fitting an old man who doesn't have enough strength to even sit up by himself for a prosthetic!" Again, the question seemed to confound the young caregiver and he repeated; "Because it was ordered by a doctor and Medicare will cover it." I quickly realized that further conversation was pointless. Luckily my father had medical power of attorney for my grandfather. He quickly told this young man that we did not agree to this and he was to leave the room while he could still walk without a prosthetic himself.

This is a very small example of a much larger issue. The question is how do we address these situations in a caring, compassionate way that provides good care to the elderly, but without so much unnecessary spending? In my opinion, the solution could be found in the proposed enhanced role of the RUC. In addition to coverage policies and care pathways, the RUC could be charged with creating coverage policies for end-of-life care. Like the other coverage policies, we would still have an appeal process for those cases that don't fit the standard guidelines.

Under this model, the experience that we had with my grandfather would have never happened. In his case, the request for a prosthetic would have been denied because of a coverage policy that would include things like the patient's strength and projected ability to ambulate with the prosthetic. This approach could also be used in some of the very expensive beginning-of-life decisions involving what care should be provided for premature infants with extremely poor prognoses.

If this approach produced just a 10% savings in end-of-life costs for Medicare, it would mean over $15 billion saved per year. I tend to think that the actual savings would be significantly more, but $15 billion is nothing to sneeze at.

LEGAL REFORMATION

Another place we should look for savings, though not specifically related to rationing, is tort reform. Everyone in the industry agrees that "defensive medicine" exists. The challenge is to determine its impact on the cost of healthcare and then find a way to eliminate it. In 2014, a study lead by the Cleveland Clinic was published in the *Journal of the American Medical Association* that examined defensive medicine and its financial impact. The study noted that 28% of the 4,200 physician orders studied were at least "somewhat" defensive and 2.9% were "entirely" defensive. The Cleveland Clinic study estimated the annual cost of defensive medicine to be $46 billion dollars per year. There are other studies, not to mention the American Medical Association itself, that put the cost significantly higher. For now, though, let's use the conservative Cleveland Clinic number of $46 billion.

Tests and services performed for defensive reasons don't have any real clinical value, they don't change the course of treatment. With this in mind, we begin to understand just how staggering that $46 billion figure really is. To help put it into perspective, $46 billion is about the annual revenue of companies like FedEx and Disney. That's how much money we're wasting on defensive medicine, all to keep the lawsuits at bay. That doesn't even include the cost of malpractice carriers defending frivolous lawsuits or the actual malpractice payouts. In 2013, there were $3.7 billion dollars in malpractice payouts.

Finding good data on the cost of defending cases is difficult. However, I did speak with an executive at a large medical malpractice carrier who told me his company spent more money successfully defending cases where no additional money was awarded than they did in all of their payouts for losing cases put together. The reason is because in states without tort reform, patients and their attorneys have an incentive to go for a malpractice "home run." The potential for a lottery-like payoff creates incentives for large numbers of baseless malpractice claims and expensive defense in court.

A perfect example of this comes from my own state of North Carolina. Former presidential candidate John Edwards made a fortune on medical malpractice cases. His specialty was suing hospitals and obstetricians for causing cerebral palsy during delivery. A 2008

CNSnews story titled *"Did 'Junk Science' Make John Edwards Rich?"* detailed Mr. Edward's use of emotion rather than science to convince juries to make large awards to his clients. In a comprehensive analysis of Edwards' legal career by *The Boston Globe* in 2003, it was said Edwards' trial summaries " . . . routinely went beyond a recitation of his case to a heart-wrenching plea to jurors to listen to the unspoken voices of injured children." The *Globe* cited an example of Edwards' oratorical skills from a medical malpractice trial in 1985. Edwards had alleged a doctor and a hospital had been responsible for the cerebral palsy afflicting then five-year-old Jennifer Campbell:

> "I have to tell you right now—I didn't plan to talk about this— right now I feel her (Jennifer), I feel her presence," Edwards told the jury according to court records. "[Jennifer's] inside me and she's talking to you . . . And this is what she says to you. She says, 'I don't ask for your pity. What I ask for is your strength. And I don't ask for your sympathy, but I do ask for your courage.'"

Edwards' emotional plea worked. Jennifer Campbell's family won a record jury verdict of $6.5 million against the hospital where the girl was born—a judgment reduced later to $2.75 million on appeal. Edwards also settled with Jennifer's obstetrician for $1.5 million.

This is exactly the problem that tort reform will help eliminate. If we remove the ability to award non-compensatory damages, it eliminates these kinds of "home-run" cases that are based on emotion and not science or fact. Again, it is difficult to calculate just how much money this could save, but I think it's safe to say it's a significant number.

TECHNOLOGY

Another area of potential cost savings could come from the creation of a common national electronic records format. Right now there are several physician and hospital EMR systems. While individually they work fairly well, none of them talk to each other. A recent study showed that 1 in 5 radiology tests done in a hospital was a duplicate effort and could have been avoided if the hospital had access to previous studies done elsewhere. This issue alone increases healthcare costs nationwide by over $20 billion per year.

What I propose is the creation of a common format and translation for all commercial electronic medical records. This common format would allow for an easier exchange of data and records. Secondly, I propose the creation of a common data interface and exchange system to be developed and managed by the federal government. Compliance could be achieved by offering hospitals and physicians an increase in Medicare reimbursement for being on a system that is certified as compliant with the national standards and also for connecting to the national data exchange. This would allow a hospital in Florida, for example, to see the records from a patient traveling from Texas if something happened while she was vacationing in the Sunshine State. It would also have other benefits, such as reducing prescription drug abuse, since hospital ERs could see prescriptions for that patient from other hospitals in the area—or even around the country.

The final areas we need to attack reside at the very core of insurance and how it works.

FINANCE CHANGES

The current system provides no incentive for individuals to take an active role in the financing of their healthcare. This is left entirely up to the government or their employers. The only incentive for individuals is actually a penalty through the individual mandate. One way this lack of participation can be addressed is through an expanded use of HSAs and how they're funded. My proposal follows the same overall operating premise as the 401(k) and would promote savings on healthcare expenses, patient responsibility, participation, engagement, and consumerism. These individual HSA accounts can be funded by employers, individuals, and the federal government. All federal subsidies under the current ACA formula would be deposited into the individual HSA accounts. To qualify for a subsidy, individuals must file an income tax return and must purchase health insurance. Citizens may also elect to make pre-tax deposits into their HSAs, without limitation. The individual mandate would still apply.

Individuals qualifying for the means-based subsidies have the following options:

1. Utilize subsidies to purchase health insurance through the marketplace.
2. Subsidize required employee contribution through employer group policy or individual or dependent coverage.
3. Receive the net balance of the subsidy remaining after health insurance premiums are paid, to be deposited into a taxpayer directed HSA for additional medical expenses.

Funds in the individual's HSA accounts are eligible to be used for medical expenses, *including* health insurance premiums, for the individual or his or her immediate family as defined by the Internal Revenue Service Code. HSA accounts remain active until the death of the individual, and upon death of the individual, the funds remaining in the HSA are transferred to immediate family members' HSA accounts. If left undesignated, or there are no qualified immediate family members, then funds are transferred back to the federal Medicare and Medicaid fund.

The employer mandate as currently designed would continue, with the addition of a requirement for employers to provide an employee the option to select whether to participate in the group health insurance policy or have an equal amount deposited into the employee's HSA. Employers would have the following options:

1. Provide a group policy to employees.
2. Deposit an amount for each employee equal to the cost of a Bronze plan into employees' HSAs.
3. Pay the fine related to employer mandate.

This expansion of the use of HSAs addresses one of the problems with the ACA as currently written. Currently if an employer offers qualified coverage to an employee, it removes their ability to access any federal subsidy in the exchange market. This often hurts low-income employees who would be better off if their employer didn't offer any insurance.

INSURANCE REFORM

Alain Enthoven, and almost every other economist who studies healthcare, agree that part of the problem with healthcare costs are the "free riders"—those who benefit from the U.S. healthcare safety net but don't participate in the insurance pool. In order to have an efficient insurance market, we need the vast majority—preferably all—of the people in this country to participate. The reason this is important to cost control has to do with the fundamental principle upon which insurance operates. Insurance, by definition, is the spreading of a cost over a large number of people or over a period of time. Insurance is designed to pool small amounts of money from a large number of people and then use that money to pay for the significant costs generated by a small portion of the population. This is critical in healthcare given that the top 5% of care consumers account for 50% of all healthcare spending while the healthiest 50% of the population consume less than 5% of the total. This skewness makes it critical that the healthy 50% of the population doesn't opt out of purchasing health insurance. If this happens, there is no way the other 50%, especially the top 5%, who really need it could ever afford coverage.

This problem in particular plagues the ACA and the exchange marketplaces right now. Many of the people who have joined the exchange have more clinically severe health problems, and not enough of the healthy population has been attracted to the new marketplace to offset the cost of caring for them. The healthy people are choosing to go without coverage, diminishing the revenue pool. This demonstrates why one of the most important aspects of healthcare cost control is making sure that everyone pays for some level of coverage.

The ACA's individual and employer mandates are not enough to force full, or even close to full, enrollment. This gives us another task to undertake: how do we encourage, or force, large-scale participation? I would keep the current exchanges, as I believe they create a useful marketplace for individuals who want to purchase insurance. However, I would propose the following enhancements to help support the exchanges and push for more widespread participation:

1. Pass legislation that requires all insurance companies, and those companies administering insurance-like products (i.e., self-insured plans), to also sell fully insured plans, as well as exchange plans, to individuals and small groups in every county where they offer their other products. This would mean companies like Cigna, Aetna, and United would be required to offer and sell individual and small-group policies, as well as exchange policies, everywhere they offer their self-insured products.

Simply put, if they want to sell the "good business"—large employer products—in an area, they will have to take *all* customers. This would include the small-group, individual, and exchange members. This would help give all consumers more choice.

2. Pass legislation that all small-group and individual commercial products must be community rated with rates approved by the state Department of Insurance commissioners.

3. Change the current COBRA laws to remove the premium increase for COBRA coverage. In addition, treat short-term COBRA coverage like unemployment insurance. Charge employers a small tax, then provide short-term coverage free to people who lose their job under the same rules as unemployment insurance. This coverage would extend for no more than 6 months. Studies show that 45% of the uninsured population is uninsured for fewer than 4 months. As such, this one move would solve almost half of the uninsured problem in this country by fixing the issue of the transitionally uninsured.

4. Establish a federal program to provide compensation to insurance companies that have a federally certified case management program designed to provide case management for a defined set of chronic diseases and high-cost individuals. Studies show that 5% of the population consumes 50% of all healthcare services. This proposed reform is designed to help these high-cost individuals, reduce costs overall, and incentivize insurance companies to address this issue.

5. Finally, the employer penalty for companies with more than 50 employees must be increased. Right now, it is significantly more expensive to provide health insurance for employees than it is to pay the penalty. It's a little bit like having a $5 speeding ticket. That won't deter much speeding. The individual mandate also needs to be strengthened to provide more incentive for individuals to pursue coverage.

PERSONAL ACCOUNTABILITY

The last thing that we need to address is another difficult one. We need to add some personal accountability to the process. Right now, the only lifestyle question asked when a person is enrolling in one of the ACA exchange plans is, "Do you smoke?" To my knowledge, there is no way for the carrier to check your answer, so I'm not sure why anyone who smokes would answer that question honestly. You could be an obese diabetic, eating a full box of Krispy Kreme donuts while sucking down a Big Gulp Mountain Dew for breakfast right before you drive to McDonalds for your super-sized double Quarter Pounder lunch while you enroll in the exchange and it wouldn't affect your rates one bit. Furthermore, there is no way for your insurance carrier to change your rates once they find out about your unhealthy and potentially expensive lifestyle. Compare this situation to auto insurance. Everyone knows and accepts that if you get four speeding tickets or a DUI, your auto insurance company is going to find out and your rates are going to increase dramatically.

We seem willing to accept the idea that we should pay more for auto insurance if we choose to drive fast or drive drunk. Insurance companies hold us financially responsible for our driving style and we agree to it largely without protest. However, we are *not* okay with the idea of paying more for health insurance if we choose to make unhealthy life style choices.

Put away the pitchforks, I'm not done.

I am not the healthiest person in the world. I am significantly over-weight and, until recently, my diet left much to be desired. I believe the ideas I have about this should apply to everyone, *including* me.

The problem with rating health insurance on lifestyle choices is it requires some exchange of information between the physician and your insurance company. This exchange opens up a whole new can of worms about privacy and how insurance companies could use that data. It's not as straightforward as auto insurance, where the police inform your insurance company after you've committed a traffic crime. The challenge will be to change our mindset from looking at rate adjustments as penalties for bad behavior to seeing them as rewards for good behavior.

Rather than increasing the rates for our overweight diabetic person, we would price everyone using community-rating guidelines, then offer premium reductions for people whose physicians certify certain healthy lifestyle choices. You're a non-smoker and your doctor certifies that every two years during your wellness visit? You get a reduction in your rates. You're not overweight and your blood pressure and cholesterol are under control? You get another discount in your rates. You *are* overweight but following a physician-monitored weight loss program? You get a discount.

You can see where I'm going with this. This would not only incentivize good behavior but also incentivize regular visits to your primary care physician, as these discounts would need to be re-certified every two years.

Since most people with insurance have it provided by their employer, though, my plan would require these discounts be given directly to the employee, and that this revenue be tax-exempt. Think about that for a minute. This would provide a direct, tax-free income incentive to the employee and their family to get involved and lead healthy lifestyles. It also helps the people who may need it most, as many studies show a direct correlation between unhealthy practices and lower income levels. The people in this category are the ones who could be most helped by this increase in income and who can have the most impact on healthcare costs through lifestyle changes. The employers win through reductions in their premium renewals as their companies become healthier, along with a reduction in workdays lost from illness and disease.

That's it, my prescription for curing our worsening condition. I don't underestimate how hard some of this would be. Many aspects of the cure are not easy, and I won't say they won't require significant changes in how things are done currently. What I will say, though, is if you don't think the ideas above are worth the effort, it's probably time to grab a stiff drink and read Chapter 8 again.

CHAPTER 10

Value-Based Reimbursement

So, some of you were probably confused when I ended the last chapter with no mention of one of the hottest catch phrases in healthcare these days: "value-based reimbursement." Well don't worry, that'd be like going through the holidays without Pumpkin Spice. I didn't include it in my prescription for a cure because the topic deserves its own chapter and I really don't think value-based reimbursement is going to be a big part of the cure. Instead, I see it as a long-term approach to "healthy living," so to speak.

Let's say our healthcare system, along with our cost problems, is like a patient who has a high risk of a fatal heart attack in the next couple years. He is overweight and has high blood pressure, severe artery blockage, and terrible cholesterol numbers. For this patient, the cure needs to be immediate and impactful. Things like surgery to clear the blockage, medication for blood pressure and cholesterol, and a pretty aggressive diet program are all prescriptions for this kind of patient. When the patient gets to a healthier state, *then* we can talk about long-term lifestyle issues like regular exercise and a heart-healthy diet.

These are the kinds of things that will keep the cardiac risk from coming back but are too slow to address the very immediate concern that an already risky patient presents. In my mind, value-based reimbursement falls in the same category. It's not immediate enough to deal with our current problems but will become critical to make sure we can maintain the cost savings we gain through the actions in the previous chapter. It'll also help ensure we never get into this position again.

The idea of value-based reimbursement is an easy one, and one that appeals to an economist like me. It's much like the concept of diet and exercise, though—easy to understand but sometimes hard to do. Our current system of reimbursing healthcare providers for the care they provide is filled with perverse incentives. Doctors and hospitals get paid for quantity—more money for more services. Ordering more tests and doing more procedures increases revenue. The doctor who sees a patient and doesn't order any tests or prescribe any medications or treatments in the current system is going to be taking home the lowest paycheck.

It's not just the revenue from the testing or the procedures. The act of ordering testing or prescribing medications or procedures can help support more complex decision making which can elevate the level of the visit and thus bring in more compensation for that visit. In addition, it can create the necessity for a follow-up visit to interpret and communicate the results of the testing that was ordered. This is what we're seeing in our current environment: the financial incentives for providers are the exact opposite of what we want. If they make all of their patients healthy, the providers go out of business.

Now I'm not saying that doctors all order unnecessary testing and do things for monetary reasons only. After 30 years in healthcare I'm still amazed at how many physicians continue to practice care for the good of the patient and at a detriment to their own bank account. Let me give you an example. I work with a neurology group that includes several pediatric neurologists. These doctors see a significant number of Medicaid patients. These patients have the greatest need but also have some of the highest "no-show" rates as well as serious compliance issues. They are also the worst-paying patients this group has because Medicaid has the lowest fee schedule.

The group's CFO did a cost accounting study that showed the Medicaid patients' revenue didn't even cover the overhead for the practice. That means that every time one of those physicians entered a room to see a Medicaid child, not only did the doctor not get paid anything, he or she actually took a financial loss. It *cost* the physician money to see a Medicaid patient.

We explained that it was as if the doctor had to reach into his or her checkbook and give the state some money for the pleasure of seeing that patient. Even with that information the group chose to continue to care for Medicaid patients because these kids needed care and there was nowhere else for them to go. I wonder how many other businesses would do that? Certainly not insurance companies.

So, if the current system has all the wrong incentives, what system should we adopt? That's the very reason for the discussion around value-based medicine or value-based reimbursement. The concept is to pay for the "value" the physician creates rather than how much he or she does. In its simplest form, it's paying doctors to keep people healthy rather than paying them for when they're sick. Sounds easy, right? So, is the concept of diet and exercise, and if that's so easy why am I, and millions of other Americans, still overweight? The answer is that it's harder than it sounds.

The first thing you need to understand about this concept is it's a little like a unicorn. Everyone knows what a unicorn *is* but no one has ever actually *seen* one. Everyone in healthcare is talking about value-based reimbursement. Whole forests have probably been sacrificed to print the presentations that have been created on this topic. Everyone knows what it is, but when you ask for large-scale examples of it *in practice*, the stammering begins. Getting the process going isn't going to be easy, nor is it going to help significantly over the next two to five years. Don't get me wrong, we still need to pursue this idea, as it's the key to our long-term success, but we shouldn't kid ourselves that this is going to fix our short-term problems.

I'm not going to go into the details of how to do this or what form it should take, because to be honest, that could—and has—filled a book by itself. Rather than go through that, I will simply say this: Physicians and hospitals need to start to prepare for this tectonic shift in how they get paid. It will require a whole new mindset and approach to your businesses. It will make things like data analysis and approaches to population health a critical part of your thinking. It will feel like you're learning a whole new language, and like learning a new language, you're going to say the wrong thing from time to time. Start preparing now, because this shift is inevitable, and as a wise man once said, "If you don't like change you are going to hate being irrelevant." That just happens to be the perfect segue into my next chapter on the new mindset.

CHAPTER 11

The New Mindset

I f we're going to address our immediate issues with healthcare costs, then move on to a more sustainable model, we need to change the historic mindset held by providers and, maybe more importantly, consumers of care. Both society in general, and the healthcare industry specifically, need to change our way of thinking and adopt a new approach.

During the past several decades, we have proven several things. We have proven that we can create a healthcare system with incredible access. Show me any other country with the kind of access and availability of world-class healthcare delivery. There isn't one. In this country, you can be diagnosed and treated with incredible quality in an amazingly short period of time.

We have also proven that we can advance the boundaries of technology in healthcare at an incredible pace. Today we take technology like MRI,s for granted. The MRI wasn't invented until 1971. The paper illustrating the invention was published in 1973 with the first clinically useful image being captured in 1980. From concept to reality, this technology was developed in fewer than 10 years. Today we have expanded the use of MRI into a critical diagnostic tool and can even use it to create 3D images of the cardiovascular system. We've shown the world that when it comes to healthcare, we can do it all.

Unfortunately, we've shown that we're going to break the bank doing it. We have proven that we can take the proverbial credit card of the wealthiest nation in the history of mankind and max it out. While we have been focused on the level of care and access we can provide, we seem to have given no thought to how we're going to pay for it all. That is how we got where we are today and that is why we need to change the way we think about healthcare.

The first change in the mindset is for everyone to start adding economics to *all* of their decision making. I know many people find that difficult to accept when we're talking about healthcare, but we have to get over that taboo. Consider the following example: One of your children needs surgery. The surgeon is excellent. Unfortunately, he is also very expensive. There is another surgeon who is half the cost of the first surgeon but statistics would suggest that your child's chance of dying from the procedure is also twice as high with this surgeon. Would you save the money and use the cheaper surgeon? Of course not, this is your child and there is no price you wouldn't pay to keep little Billy alive. So, you go with the better and more expensive surgeon and after the surgery you drive home in your 2002 Chevy Blazer, get into an accident and die.

Why did I add that last part? The 2002 Chevy Blazer had the highest mortality rate per million miles in 2002. What's also true is the 2002 Toyota 4 Runner was the 4th safest vehicle in terms of deaths per million miles in 2002. The risk of death driving a Chevy Blazer was almost 20 times more than the Toyota, but the Toyota is only 25% more expensive. So, every day, people put their children in a car that has a much higher chance of being involved in a fatal accident to save what would amount to $100 a month in a car payment.

Now I know this isn't a perfect example, but it does illustrate my point, which is this: people make decisions every day that trade health and safety for money. The problem is that we are not comfortable injecting economic or monetary factors into a healthcare decision-making process. Getting comfortable with it will be a very slow and difficult change, but it has to be done. Patients, doctors, all of us need to start embracing the new mindset of factoring economic realities into how care is provided and to whom.

Let me give you another example. Let's say that we faced a significant shortage of flu vaccine. Doctors and patients would all agree that, given a limited supply, we need to make sure the most at-risk patients get the vaccine first. These would include the elderly, children, and patients with compromised respiratory systems. If there is still supply leftover, we can use it for others. How is that different from the fact that there is a limited supply of money?

The new mindset is going to need to look more deeply at what we are providing and, as consumers, what we're demanding. In some cases, that will mean not taking advantage of new developments in technology or treatments if the increased cost isn't justified by a corresponding increase in clinical benefit. In other cases, it will be looking at less costly clinical approaches that may not be as good as another approach but, for a given patient population, are "good enough." This is a significant shift in thinking, from addressing the individual patient to the whole population of patients.

Right now, our clinical decision-making process is entrenched at the individual level. What can I do for my patient that is the very best for him or her? The problem with that thinking is it ignores the negative impact that type of behavior has on the whole population. It does this by over-utilizing limited resources on one patient and that, by the very definition of being "limited," means those resources are not available for other patients.

Another shift that needs to take place in this industry is something most other industries do every day and it has to do with the way the healthcare delivery system looks at budgets and operations. Most other industries assume that revenue is a fixed number set by market forces. For example, GM knows that they can't charge $100,000 for a basic truck. They know that product can be sold at a price range from $20,000 to $30,000. They know consumers won't pay more for this product mostly because Ford sells a similar product for that price range. So, given a fixed revenue per truck that is set by market forces,

GM knows the only way they can make profit is to figure out how to make that truck for less than $20,000. They play the cost and efficiency game, not the revenue game, because revenue is fixed by the market.

Most of the healthcare delivery model looks at things completely opposite to that model. Most healthcare providers add up the costs that they either think they need or have historically needed, then demand a price for their product or service that will produce profit levels they've set for themselves. This approach is seen in every part of healthcare delivery, from physicians to hospitals and, of course, to drug companies. When was the last time you saw Wall Street get all excited because a pharmaceutical company was devoting significant resources to more efficient production capabilities? Never. They get excited by the money put into R&D because they know no matter what it costs to produce that next wonderful drug, the drug company will be able to set a price well above its cost and produce wonderful *profit*.

Many reasons and economic factors have produced this situation in healthcare. We've discussed some of them, and dwelling on them isn't useful. We need to change and start treating healthcare like other industries. Healthcare providers need to start looking at revenue as fixed and then work on how to produce their product such that it can be profitable at that level.

Let's take the simplest example. Say we have a physician group that is going to get $100 for every patient visit. The problem is that when they add up their costs, they come up with $125 per visit, fully loaded. It doesn't take an Ivy League MBA to know that if costs exceed revenues you don't have a very sustainable business model. So, how do they get their costs down below $100 per visit? This involves doing things that other businesses have done for years. They look at what drives their costs and examine how they could do things more efficiently.

In healthcare, simple things like adding NPs (Nurse Pratitioners) or PAs (Physician Assistants) to see some of a practice's patients will help because they're less expensive than a doctor. Using MAs (Medical Assistants) instead of RNs (Registered Nurses) as clinical support will help. Look at support staffing and internal processes to see if you can eliminate inefficiencies and reduce costs. All of these are basic business practices in almost every other industry, but it we are being honest, are rarely *if ever* fully explored in healthcare. More advanced efficiency efforts are almost never seen.

For example, the practice in our example has a significant fixed cost for their facility. They have to pay the same rent or mortgage if they are open five hours a day, five days a week, or ten hours a day, seven days a week. So, let's say they are open eight hours a day, five days a week. Staying open another two hours a day, or opening for five hours one day on the weekend, would reduce their fixed facility cost per visit by 25%. This in itself could be the difference between being profitable or not, not to mention it could potentially increase patient satisfaction.

This approach is not easy and not without its challenges. Increasing your capacity by being open more means finding staff and physicians to work those hours and, in some cases, can be a significant change in lifestyle. I understand the challenges this presents. However, let's keep in mind that factories have been running three shifts for decades. They don't run three shifts because a huge number of people really want to work from 11 p.m. to 7 a.m. every day. They do it because in many cases it is the only way to survive and produce their product at a competitive price. I don't think we need to turn our healthcare facilities into three-shift factories, but I think there's significant work that can and must be done to produce healthcare services more efficiently, and it's imperative that we begin that work now.

The final mindset shift is going to sound like something a consultant thought up (and probably did), who went on to make a pile of money talking about without producing any tangible results (and many consultants probably have and continue to): putting the patient, and the population, in the center of healthcare delivery. Patient- and Population-Centered Care is the kind of consultant speak that makes me think of buzzwords like paradigm shifting, transformative, outside of the box thinking, collaborative synergistic . . . ok, I'm done.

What I *am* talking about is not some difficult-to-define, easy-to-put-on-a-PowerPoint slide concept, but rather a concrete shift in thinking. It's an approach where the delivery system puts more focus on the patient as a customer who needs to be attracted to the business rather than a given. In the world ahead, this kind of mindset will become more and more critical. Things like extended hours, flexible scheduling, and expanded use of technology are all areas where the healthcare delivery system can and should become more patient and service focused.

Think about this for a second: I can book a flight online, check in online, and use my phone as my boarding pass. Why do I have to sign several paper forms every time I go to my doctor? This shift in mindset is good not only for attracting and keeping patients, it will also help with things like compliance and patient loyalty.

My last comment on the need for this shift in patient focus is this: right now, most medical practices' hours, scheduling, and operational efficiency issues work best for people without busy schedules and day-to-day time commitments. That describes the unemployed, those on Medicare, and Medicaid. Those happen to be the worst-paying patients most physicians treat. My point here is that no one else would set up a business that only worked for people who couldn't pay for the service.

CHAPTER 12

Summary and Conclusions

The US healthcare system is a product of who we are and what we are as a country. It's a combination of a nation that is blessed with prosperity that the rest of the world can only envy, combined with a very generous people who time and time again open their hearts to help those in need. It's influenced by an economic environment and a "no challenge is too big" culture that has pioneered many of the most amazing technological advancements in history. It is without a doubt the very best healthcare delivery system in the world . . . if you can afford it.

The problem with our healthcare delivery system is the same problem we have in other areas, like our federal deficit. We are nation that doesn't have a very good track record of fiscal responsibility. We have close to a $20 trillion national debt, yet we are the first country to give aid to another country in need. We will extend benefits to our own citizens, the elderly, the poor, the unemployed, when we don't seem to have an ability to finance those commitments. Heck, we're the country that invented the term "unfunded mandate" to describe the commitments we've made to our elderly in the forms of Social Security and Medicare. We will even extend benefits to people who are not our citizens and are in this country illegally.

This is what makes us a great nation, but it can make us the victim of our own charity and fiscal irresponsibility. How many nations sent us money after the housing crash of 2008? How much money did China send the United States to help all those people who lost their homes, jobs, or retirement? Many countries sent us thoughts and prayers after 9/11 but did any send money to help rebuild New York? I'm not asking for other countries to fix our financial problems; I'm pointing out that there is some truth to the statement that charity begins at home.

I'm happy we are a charitable people. I hope we never lose that about our country. It's truly what makes us great. The fact that U.S. soldiers were on the beaches in Normandy and that our hearts and checkbooks are extended to those in need both inside and outside our borders is what makes us who we are, and we need to protect that. In protecting that American quality, we also need to realize that, just like the housing crisis of 2008, if healthcare melts down, no one *else* is going to help *us*. No one is going to send billions of dollars to make sure our citizens get the care they need or help us with the incredible unemployment that will result. We are in this alone and we alone need to fix our problem.

The problem is daunting, the challenges great, and the decisions difficult. If it were easy we would have already done it. However, the consequences of doing nothing are much worse. This is one can that we can't afford to kick down the road. Compared to the housing crisis, a meltdown in healthcare will be like cancer compared to the flu.

It is clear to me that we need to act and it needs to happen now. Blindly following the same trail we've been on for the last 50 years is going to result in some very unpleasant results when this market makes its own adjustment.

We can await our fate or we can blaze a new trail.